She's Expecting Multiples

A guide for the friends & family of those expecting twins, triplets and more

Sharlene Gittens-Francis

Dedication

To my children Kalicia, Kaylene and Kevin you have made carrying triplets worth it!

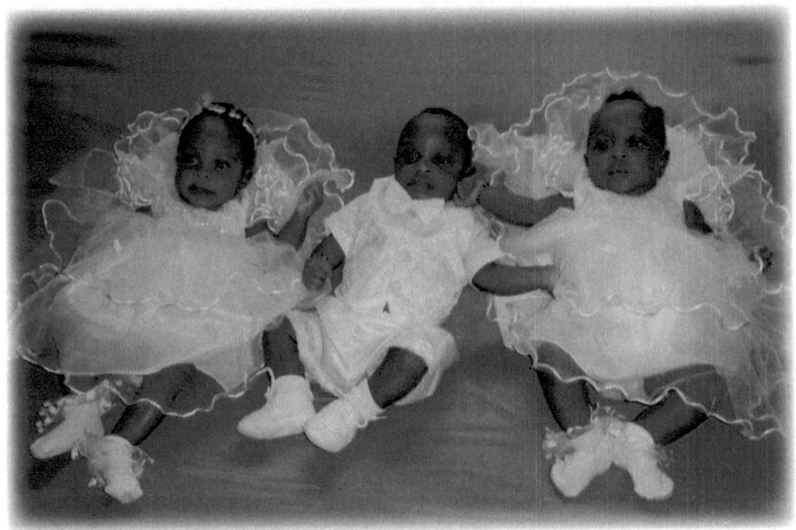

To my late grandmother who sadly did not get to enjoy her great grandchildren for as long as we hoped and as long as she would have desired.

Acknowledgements

Thanks to all our family members and friends who have helped and are helping us along the way, especially my mother, father, sister, mother-in-law and father-in-law. I also want to thank my husband and friends who saw this book's potential when it was merely an idea and scribbles on paper, whose comments and ideas have been incorporated in helping me gather and package my message, and who have pushed me to get this book finished. I appreciate all those mothers of multiples and their helpers who have made this book possible with their input, experiences, strategies and ideas. I also wish to thank the online communities, blogs, chat groups and Facebook groups that tolerated my questions and surveys while I was on my information quest.

Note from the Author

Dear reader,

Being pregnant and giving birth to my triplets has been the single most life changing moment in my existence. I have learned and continue to learn so much from it about myself and the people around me. I would never wish this experience away. Many of my friends and relatives felt helpless when I told them I was expecting multiples, but they quickly got with the program. I can attest that the key to my happy, stress free, successful multiple pregnancy was thanks to the help and thoughtfulness of my friends and family.

If you have a friend or a relative or even a mere acquaintance who is expecting multiples i.e. twins, triplets or more, you can be part of this life changing experience for them. I will show you the valuable assistance that you can render and give you a better idea of how and when to approach her. I have also used my experiences and that of other mothers of multiples, to give you a better understanding of what your friend/relative is or will be going through from an emotional, social, medical, physical and financial perspective.

Think about it. The flutter of the heartbeats on the ultrasound machine and the health of the babies growing inside of her can be attributed to something that you have done. Just imagine that the pride and jubilation she feels on the delivery of her sweet bundles of joy will be attributed to your help and invaluable contributions.

Sharlene Gittens-Francis

Table of Contents

Preface

Among the doctor's orders to rest, relax and eat healthy, I have discovered the way to have a happy, healthy multiple pregnancy is through the invaluable help of people like you. Friends and relatives can make this experience more manageable and less overwhelming. I found the efforts of my friends and relatives helped me avoid stress, exhaustion, anxiety and more importantly preterm labor and I wish the same for your friend/relative. Fortunately, I managed to carry my triplets to 36+ weeks.

There are many books on the market for expectant parents of multiples, particularly expectant mothers, on the various aspects of multiple pregnancies. All of them mention these parents should get help while she is pregnant, when the babies arrive or both. However, these books fail to explain how to go about getting this help.

The love, support and help that I got from my friends and family during my pregnancy inspired me to write this book. I created this book to help you, those that care enough to want to use their skills and talents to help the expectant mother of multiples (MoM)--have a happy, healthy and successful pregnancy. This book will:

- Help you to understand the situations that your friend or relative are facing or may face
- Give you ideas of questions you can ask (or not) to understand her situation
- Equip you with the knowledge to make a valuable contribution to her situation
- Give you ideas of what you can do to assist her

- Quell the helpless feeling you may feel when you hear that your friend or relative is expecting multiples
- Give you tips on topics relevant to her unique situation like shopping, space considerations, must haves, bed rest
- Help you fulfill your desire to be a good friend and bring smiles to the faces of people you care about

I wrote this book when I could breathe again after my babies turned one year. Luckily for me, I still have my friends and relatives chipping in. This gave me the opportunity to educate more people about how they can help make carrying and raising multiples easier and our new lives less daunting.

The acronym MoM and PoM is used to refer to the mother of multiples and parents of multiples respectively throughout this book.

The views in this book are my personal opinions and do not replace the advice of medical practitioners, psychologists or religious authority. This book is designed to give you an idea of what an expectant MoM will experience during her pregnancy as well as how you can pitch in to make it a more bearable and enriching experience. You are free to agree or disagree and perform the activities or not as suits your personality, lifestyle, preference and relationship with the expectant PoM.

This book shares helpful tips and simple strategies to make the day to day situations and circumstances of the expectant PoMs more manageable. Let it be your guide. Help them successfully move on to the next exciting period of their life - **Raising Multiples!**

What's in this Book

This book gives some insight into what the expectant MoM is or may soon be facing. It will walk you through the various aspects of her pregnancy from an emotional, social, medical, physical and financial perspective. I have organized this book to make it easy for you to understand what your friend or relative is going through, answer some of your questions about multiple births, have conversations with her without offending her, give meaningful proactive assistance and give you ideas to help her relax and have fun while pregnant. It explains my personal experience with my triplet pregnancy and also provides a general idea of what your friend/ relative may be experiencing based on what I have read, been told by my network of MoMs and mothers of singletons. To help give you a wider perspective I conducted a few informal surveys, and participated in online and actual conversations (i) in my network of parents of multiples **(Survey: Fun being pregnant with multiples - Is it or isn't it?)** and (ii) on their friends and relatives and my friends and relatives **(Survey of present and prospective helpers to MoMs). - See Appendix 1: Gathering Perspectives.**

As a mother of triplets, experience has shown me that we don't always know what we need and we may feel it will threaten our independence if we ask for help. In retrospect, I realize that we need someone who:

- Understands our situation
- Knows how to engage us in meaningful conversations
- Anticipates our needs and pro-actively offers assistance
- Makes valuable contributions at the right time

There is little that you can control during her pregnancy. However, you can keep her on that less stressful road of having a happy successful pregnancy with some simple thoughtful gestures. This book identifies some priceless ways to help her on that journey.

I have included some other relevant information like tips for shopping,

Priceless ways to help an expectant MoM

Emotionally	- Understand their situation - Give emotional support - Know what to say (or not) to the expectant MoM - Help with researching and networking
Socially	- Engage her in fun and relaxing activities - Help her with her other children - Plan and organise a baby shower
Physically	- Promote healthy eating habits - Be a helpful substitute - Do chores and run errands
Physical Appearance	- Assist with maternity shopping - Pamper her
Financially	- Kick start the baby shopping - Give a financial contribution - Source cost savings
Other	- Help during bed rest or hospitalisation - Plan and organise as the due date comes close

baby showers, and questions on her mind to name a few. I have also utilized a few icons for easier reading:

From my triplet
pregnancy experience

Best ways to help the
expectant MoM

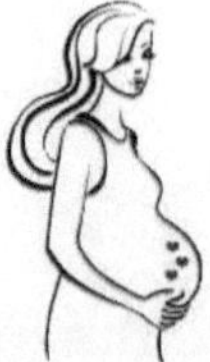

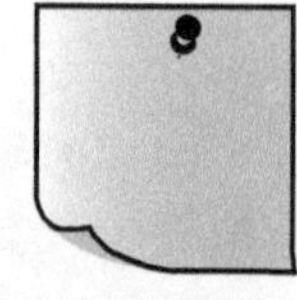

Quotes from expectant
PoMs or MoMs

Multiples facts

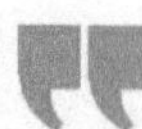

There are over 150 activities listed in this book that you can use to help her along the road to a happy, successful pregnancy. Some don't cost a thing, some take little effort, and some are quite simple. There are also others that may require time, energy, thought and of course money. You can choose activities to match your situation.

You can be that person! You can help the expectant MoM make it through these next few months relatively stress free. It is extremely easy. Just peruse this book and take my experience and explanations into consideration and adopt a few activities and pointers. Utilize them and you will be considered the most perceptive and thoughtful friend or relative!

1

Introduction

So, you've gotten the news, now what?

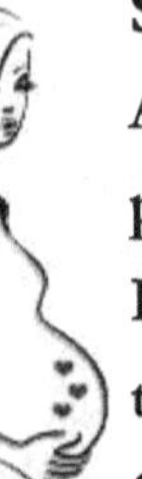

Shared Excitement

A few months ago, my best friend told me she was pregnant. I was so happy for her and her husband. I asked her if she knew the sex of the baby and she told me it was a surprise.

One day we went shopping for baby clothes and gear and I picked up a pink blanket and a blue blanket. With a wink, hoping she would reveal to me her guarded secret I asked, "Which do you want a blue or a pink?"

She responded, "I will need another pink as well!"

- Best friend of expectant mother of triplets

So, you have just found out that your sister, sister-in-law, close friend or relative is pregnant with multiples and she is only a few months into her pregnancy. I cannot imagine the wave of emotion that you are feeling. But as a mother of triplets I can surely relate to her rush of emotions when she got her news!

The road to delivery is a bumpy ride, starting from the day the expectant MoM gets the life changing news about her multiple pregnancy. Anxiety is heightened, her hormones are flowing and the countdown to the delivery date has begun. She has a lot of work to do to get through the next few months - preparing herself mentally, preparing for sleep deprivation, purchasing and organizing baby and mommy related paraphernalia, planning and setting up her home for the babies' arrival, preparing her marriage and other family members including pets and preparing for the post-partum period, just to name a few! She has to get her Mind, Body, House, Pocket/ Finances and Family ready for this life changing experience. The world is fascinated by multiple births and her world is going to change more than she can ever imagine. She is going to be part of a unique group of mothers who are lucky enough to carry and give birth to more than one baby at a time. You, as her close friend or relative, will be there to share in her experience, which I guarantee, will be one like no other.

Our initial reaction

I laid there waiting with bated breath to confirm what my home pregnancy test told me. I was feeling a little anxious because my husband and I had discussed having a baby for a very long time. After years of putting it off for reasons of business, studying, work, wanting a social life and all other reasons, we decided

to move on to another phase in our lives - parenthood.

I saw a puzzled look on the face of my OB/GYN as he adjusted his ultrasound machine and started to poke around some more. The doctor pushed the ultrasound machine in my direction for me to have a look. He smiled and said, "Oh how nice, I see two here! Congratulations!"

I looked at my husband in disbelief. "Did he say two?"

My husband was all smiles and, as he leaned over to hold my hand, I heard the Doc in his usual joking manner say, "Can you imagine if I saw another?" Then I saw another puzzled look on the Doc's face for a few seconds, and then he shouted, "Oh, there is another!"

There was silence. I looked at my husband unable to muster up a comment or reaction. He was smiling from ear to ear and giving the thumbs up gesture! I went numb. I had no words, no thoughts, and no reaction. For a woman who always had a snide remark or comment about everything, for once I had none. I've heard about it, I've read about it, but never ever thought about it for myself. I'm pregnant with triplets!

 - Author

The moment that you find out that you are carrying multiples will be forever embossed in your mind! Whether you had fertility treatment done, you are part of a twin, your sister has triplets or a distant cousin has sextuplets, I can tell you this - nothing can prepare you for the news of being pregnant with multiples!

Let's backtrack for a minute. Put yourself in your friend or relative's shoes. What would your reaction be if you were told that you were expecting twins? Shock? Horror? Jubilation? Excitement? What about if you were told you were expecting triplets? Does your reaction change?

There is surely a broad spectrum of reactions you can have! Especially as the number of babies that you are expecting increases. The reaction of expectant PoMs ranges from shock to numbness, excitement, disbelief and worry just to name a few! I have heard of uncontrollable laughter, use of expletives in the examination room and an instance where one horrified woman even ran out of the room in her gown! One thing is for sure though; life as you know it will be different from this point onwards. But dealing with the immediate news is just the first step. After you get this, what will you need to do from this point onwards?

2

Twins, Triplets!
How did that happen?

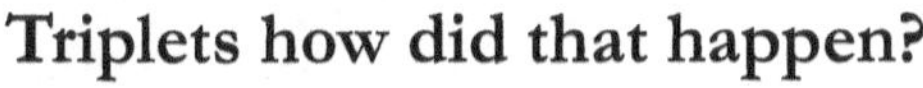

Triplets how did that happen?
When I found out that I was carrying triplets, I started to rummage through my family tree, the internet and books looking for an explanation and to get information on every possible aspect of multiple births. Suddenly, everywhere I turned I was either seeing or hearing about multiple births, more commonly twins. At the mall, in the restaurant, at the park, even in celebrity gossip!
- Author

You probably have a lot of questions about multiple births, the cause and the incidence of it. I know my friends and family did. Let me fill you in on some common questions and responses on multiple births that relatives and friends of PoMs indicated to me that they would like answers for and some facts that MoMs would like you to know. This will eliminate the need to ask some of the questions that PoMs find silly, personal or even annoying.

How common is this occurrence?

According to 2018 CDC (Center for Disease Control and Prevention) statistics, there were 3,791,712 live births in the US of which 3.3%, or 127,061 were multiple births.

US Multiples Birth Rate
Twins - 33 per 1,000 total births

Triplets and HOMs - 93 per 100,000 total births

CDC stats 2018

What are these groups of babies called?

- The following list gives the type of multiple births by number of babies involved in the pregnancy.

1- singleton	quads)	7- septuplets
2- twins	5- quintuplets (or	8- octuplets
3- triplets	quints)	9- nonuplets
4- quadruplets (or	6- sextuplets	10- decaplets

- Higher order multiples (HOMs) or super twins refer to more than two babies being born together.
- Higher order multiples can be any combination of identical or fraternal twins.

Are multiple births on the rise?

Believe it or not, the rate is declining!

- **Twin birth rate -** The US twinning rate (births in twin deliveries per 1,000 total births) rose 76% from 1980 to 2009 (from 18.9 to 33.2 per 1,000), was generally stable from 2009 through 2012, and then rose for 2013 and 2014. The 2014 rate of 33.9 was the highest ever reported. In 2018 the twin birth rate was 32.6 twins per 1,000 births, a 2% decline from the 2017 rate of 33.3.

- **Triplet and Higher Order Multiples (HOMs) birth rate -** In the US, this rate rose more than 400 percent during the 1980s and 1990s but has declined since 1998. There was 93.0 per 100,000 births for 2018, an 8% decline from 2017 (101.6) and down 52% from the 1998 peak (193.5).

- The rate in 2013 declined to 119 per 100,000 births. This is the lowest reported since 1995.

- The pronounced rise in multiple birth rates during the 1980s and 1990s has been associated with the older maternal age and the expanded use of fertility-enhancing therapies. The recent decline

US live births statistics 2014-2018

	2014	2015	2016	2017	2018
Total # of births	3988076	3978497	3945875	3855500	3791712
# of live singleton births	3848214	3841219	3810149	3723273	3664651
# of live multiple births	139862	137278	135726	132176	127061
# of twin births	135336	133155	131723	128310	123536
# of triplet births	4233	3871	3755	3675	3400
# of quadruplet births:	246	228	217	143	115
# of quintuplet and other HOMs	47	24	31	48	10

CDC stats 2014-2018

in triplet and HOMs birth rates has been associated with practice guidelines from the American Society for Reproductive Medicine intended to reduce the incidence of higher-order multiple gestation pregnancies.

Twin facts

- There are two basic types of twins: monozygotic, commonly referred to as identical twins and dizygotic, referred to as fraternal twins.

- Identical Twins vs. Fraternal Twins

  • Chances of having identical twins are 4 in 1000. This has remained the same throughout history, anywhere in the world!

  • Chances of having fraternal twins in the world is 22.8 in 1000 according to Twins magazine. However, this rate varies with factors like location, maternal age, personal history among others.

  • There is a greater possibility of fraternal twins than identical twins based on the above stats!

Identical vs. fraternal twins	
Identical twins	**Fraternal twins**
World Birth rate: 4 in 1000	World Birth rate: 22.8 in 1000
Developed from one fertilized egg	Developed from two eggs
Egg divides into two individuals who will share all their genes in common	Separate eggs, each fertilized by separate sperm
Are genetic clones of each other	Have their own unique genes
Are always the same sex	May be the same sex or opposite
Handprints and footprints are similar, but the fingerprints are different	They are no more alike than genetic single-birth brothers and sisters
Have identical features, eye and hair color	May appear similar or look completely different, may have different hair and eye colors, may be different sizes

Do twins "skip a generation"?

- Many people believe that twins "skip a generation." Twinning is passed on as a genetic trait and appears in the women only. If you are a female and your mother had fraternal twins, you would have an increased chance of having fraternal twins yourself. Your brothers would not have an increased chance of having fraternal twins themselves, but they may pass the genetic trait on to their daughters who would then have an increased chance of having twins. This makes it appear that twins skip a generation.

Do twins run in your family?

- It is the woman's ovulation pattern alone that determines whether a woman can have twins or not. Some women are naturally prone to producing more than one egg during ovulation and hence more likely to have twins and higher order multiples. It does not matter how many fraternal twins, triplets or other multiples that the male's family may have!

Did she have fertility treatment or drugs to have multiples?

- It is well known that fertility treatments can cause multiple births. This affects mainly the rate of fraternal or dizygotic twins. Also, the success of Assisted Reproductive Technology (ART) e.g. in vitro fertilization (IVF), has produced more viable embryos contributing to multiple births. However, there are many other factors that can contribute to the incidence of multiple births.

What other factors affect the incidence of multiple births?

- **Oral contraceptives** - A woman's chances increase if she conceives in the first month after discontinuing birth control pills

- **Family history** - Fraternal twins tend to run in families. Most identical twins happen by "chance" and can happen to anyone. Some women inherit the gene for hyper ovulation - the predisposition to produce multiple eggs in a single cycle
- **Race** - Africans have a higher rate while Asians have the lowest rate
- **Maternal Age** - The older one is, the higher one's chances
- **Nutrition** - Being well nourished increases the chances of multiple births, but the rates drop off with malnutrition
- **Number of previous pregnancies** - The more pregnancies you have had, the greater are your chances to conceive twins with each successive birth
- **Geographic location** - e.g. For the years 2008 to 2010, in the United States, Massachusetts, New Jersey and Connecticut reported the highest proportion of twins, while Nebraska, New Jersey, and North Dakota had the highest level of triplets and higher order births.
- **Season** - In the Northern region, most fraternal twins are conceived in July, fewest are in January, while Southern regions have more births in October or November. This is thought to be due to the length of daylight on the secretion of Follicle Stimulating Hormones.
- **Interesting fact** - Nigeria has the highest rate of twinning in the world, 1 in 22. Many scientists believe this is attributable to yams, the main staple of their diet. Yams contain a high level of a substance similar to the hormone estrogen which is thought to bring on multiple ovulations.

Why do so many celebrities have twin offspring?

In March 2014, actor Chris Hemsworth joined the fraternity of celebrities with twin offspring when he welcomed twin boys into the world. In May 2014, Swiss tennis ace Roger Federer defied the odds to become a father to twins for the second time. The two boys were born almost five years after the arrival of their twin sisters. So why do so many famous people have twin offspring? There is no proven answer to the cause of the frequency of multiples among celebrities, however the following can be noted:

- Many celebrities frequently postpone pregnancy during peak career years, as such the older maternal age makes them more prone to producing twins and other multiples than the population at large

- Multiple births are more likely to occur in pregnancies encouraged by the use of fertility drugs, often used by those waiting until later in life to pursue parenthood.

- While some celebrities try to maintain secrecy about their relationships and pregnancy, official quotes and rumors indicate that many of them have used fertility treatments. For instance Celine Dion, while others have gone on the record to indicate that they have conceived their twins naturally, for example Jennifer Lopez.

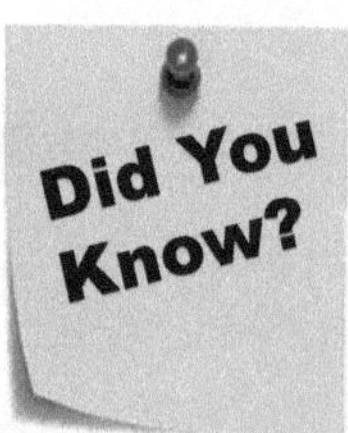

Multiples & Celebrities

Famous mothers of twins
Angelina Jolie
Celine Dion
Cybill Shepherd
Holly Hunter
Jennifer Lopez
Joan Lunden
Julia Roberts
Lisa Marie Presley
Marcia Cross
Mariah Carey
Rebecca Romijn
Sarah Jessica Parker

Famous fathers of twins
Brad Pitt
Charlie Sheen
Chris Hemsworth
Dennis Quaid
Denzel Washington
Marc Anthony
Matthew Broderick
Mel Gibson
Michael J. Fox
Patrick Dempsey
Ray Romano
Roger Federer

Famous twins
Aaron and Shawn Ashmore
Benji and Joel Madden
Dylan and Cole Sprouse
Jenna and Barbara Bush
Mary-Kate and Ashley Olsen
Tia and Tamera Mowry
Tiki and Ronde Barber

Did you know that they had a less famous twin?
Ashton Kutcher
Scarlett Johansson
Kiefer Sutherland
Vin Diesel
Gisele Bundchen
Jill Hennessy
Jon Heder
Alanis Morisette

3

What's it like carrying multiples?

Really tell me, what's it like?

It is natural to want to know how it feels to carry more than one baby at a time. I have had men and women, mothers and even children ask me this! Just to satisfy my natural curiosity I asked my network of MoMs about their needs, concerns and activities during their pregnancy with their multiples and to give an overall rating of their experience. My survey, **"Fun being pregnant with multiples - Is it on isn't it?"** was administered online to 100 MoMs of twins, triplets or quadruplets.

MoM's Pregnancy Experience

Approximately half of the MoMs surveyed indicated that they had an overall positive experience when they were pregnant with their multiples. More importantly, more than half of these MoMs thought that this was the best experience ever!

Just imagine only a few of them (15%) described the overall experience as being a negative one. One MoM even indicated that it was the worst experience ever, but she would do it again!

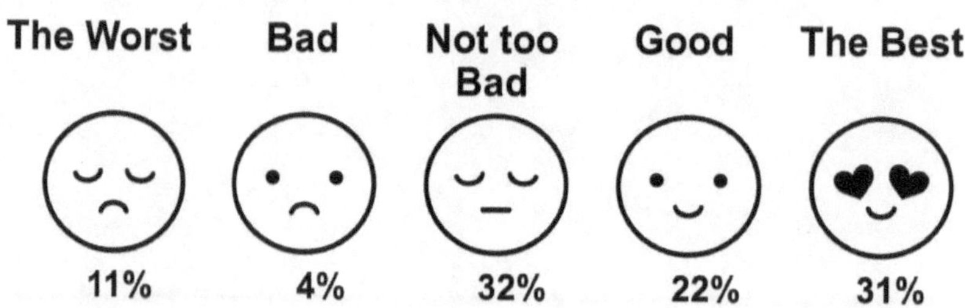

Source: Fun being pregnant with multiples – Is it or isn't it

Personally, my experience was a good one. If blessed with the opportunity to carry multiples again I would embrace it. However, I can assure you that I will not voluntarily go through that experience again. Before reading this book, h**ow did you think the experience would be if you were pregnant with twins, triplets or even more?**

In this book we will look at some of the emotional, social, physical, medical and financial matters that contribute to the overall experience of carrying multiples.

Can't wait to read the book? Here is a sneak peek of what's it like to carry multiples.

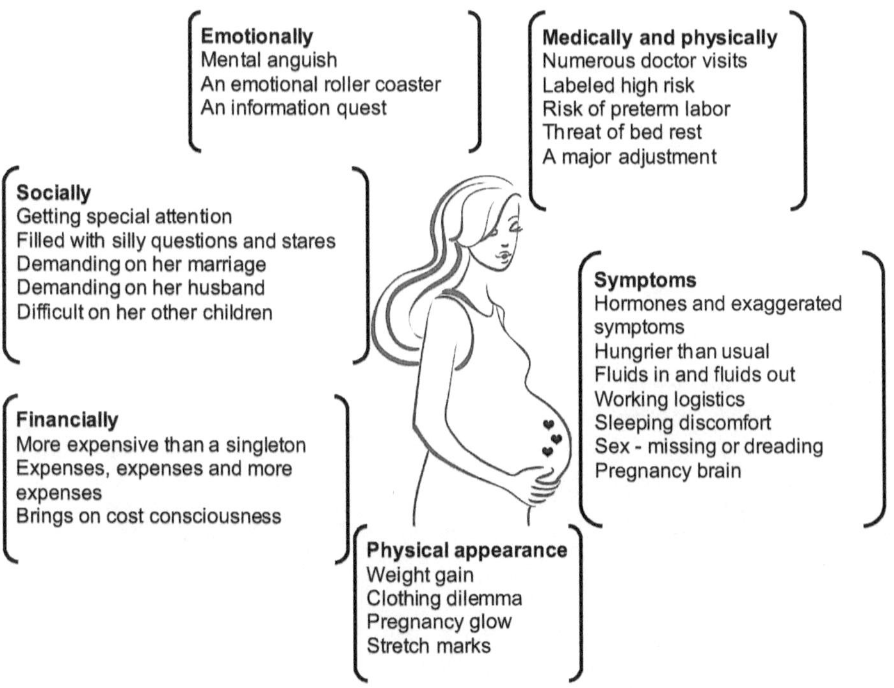

4

What can I do to help?
Extra hands needed?

Regardless of who you are, your age, life stage or profession there are loads of things you can do to assist the expectant MoM. It can be a large gesture or an exceedingly small act of kindness. I can guarantee that it will be greatly appreciated.

Every little effort helps. It will definitely help the expectant PoMs through this difficult period. It will help them have a relatively less stressful life, knowing that they have support to perform the mission for which they have been chosen.

People relate easier to people with similar experiences or who are sensitive to their present issues and state of mind. Since you probably may have no interest in joining your friend/relative in the multiple birth lanes, my advice to you is to understand or at least have an idea of what she is going through. Be on alert for indicators that she feels uncomfortable, that you are overstepping or being intrusive during your conversations and actions. Also, if she rejects your assistance be cautious and patient with her as she may be apprehensive and doubtful about the value of the help that others can provide.

Most common offers of assistance to MoM
- **Emotional support**
- **Financial assistance - monetary contribution**
- **Financial assistance - useful products**
  - **Babysitting**
  - **Assistance with chores**
  - **Meal preparation**

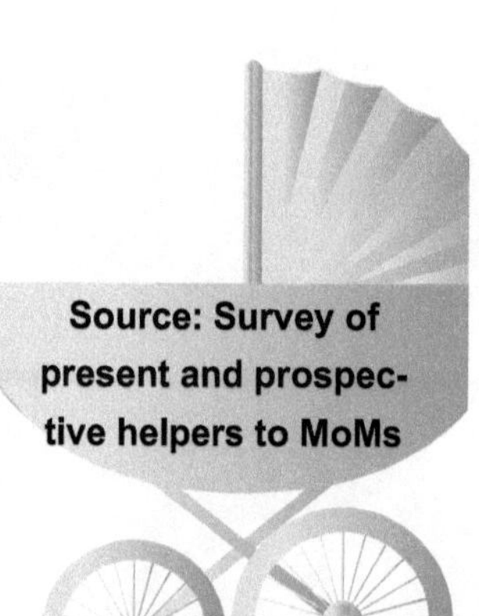

Source: Survey of present and prospective helpers to MoMs

STEPS to help the expectant MoM

Here are some simple steps to go about helping your friend or relative:

Determine her needs	- Read this book with the mission of understanding what she is going through during her pregnancy - Read **Twins, Triplets, How did that happen!** (Chapter 2, page 19) This will answer some of the initial questions about multiple births. - Ask meaningful questions with the purpose of understanding her situation - Listen to the expectant MoM and observe her situation to determine what she needs and where you can chip in - Ask if she needs anything specific; this is easier than trying to figure it out
Assess your situation	- Think about what you may need if you were pregnant with multiples. It may not be the same but it will help you empathize - Read the activities associated with the **Priceless ways to help an expectant MoM** (Page 13) identified in the next few chapters. - Assess your skills, talents, time, hobbies, finances and tolerances!
Just do it!	- Choose some activities based on her needs and your ability and constraints - Have fun doing them!

Examples or Offers to Assist

I was so scared for her to do anything more than rest and eat. I did some of her household chores, cooked, brought food, helped set up the nursery and kept her house in order when she went to the hospital.
- Mother of expectant MoM

I had to keep my sister looking good during her pregnancy. I styled her hair and gave her manicures and pedicures. She had a little difficulty reaching her toes.
- Sister of expectant MoM

They had so many questions during her pregnancy, I advised them on the risks, the Neonatal Intensive Care Unit experience and precautions to take.
- Neonatologist, relative of expectant PoMs.

I would go across and wash her car whenever I had a free moment - **Neighbor**

I was tired of seeing the yoga pants and big jerseys so I took her on a maternity shopping spree!
- Friend of expectant MoM/Fashionista

Those tiny baby clothes and all that baby gear. I was so excited to start shopping.
- Friend of expectant MoM/ shopaholic.

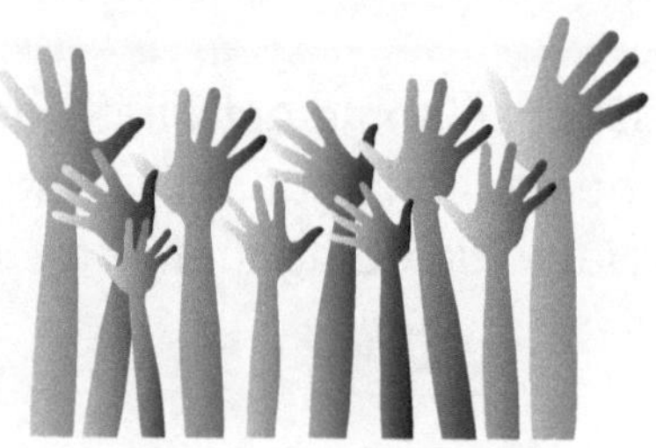

5

Emotionally
Sneak Peek

What's it like?
- **Mental anguish**
- **An emotional roller coaster**
- **An information quest**

How can I help?
- **Understand their situation**
- **Give emotional support**
- **Know what to say (or not) to the expectant MoM**
- **Help with researching and networking**

What's it like emotionally

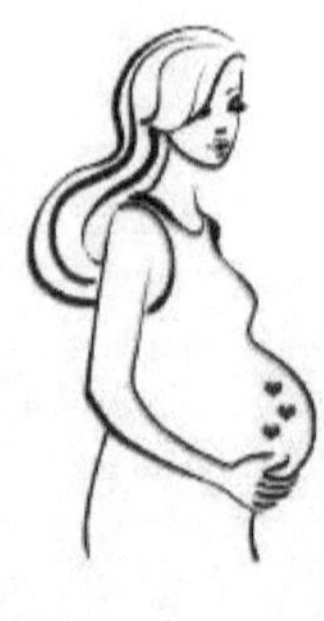

My emotionally tumultuous pregnancy

My pregnancy was a very emotional time for me. On any given day, the array of emotions I went through was unbelievable. Monitoring every twitch or pain, reading as many multiples and pregnancy related material as possible, speaking to my friends with multiples, asking my doctor tons of questions, joining online groups - all had me in a real emotional mess! I had too much information. Then there was my mother and husband aka "the movement police," constantly monitoring my every move making me feel like I was a teenager!

Excerpt from my day

<u>8:30 Excitement:</u> It is very exciting to feel my babies kick for the first time. It reinforced that everything is going to be all right.

<u>8:31 Irritated:</u> I called my husband to tell him the great news and there was no answer.

<u>9:25 Anxious:</u> It is only 16 weeks, how many more weeks to go? Should I tell everyone? Should I start shopping? Should I inform my Project Manager?

<u>10:00 Happy:</u> Went to the paint shop to choose colors for my nursery and look at some baby gear.

<u>10:45 Irritated:</u> My husband returned my call. He was not as excited as I expected by my news. His recommendation was to lie down and put my feet up.

<u>12:07 Frustrated:</u> Husband's orders, doctor's orders. I'm not used to following orders! Argh!

<u>1:14 Overwhelmed:</u> I decided to do a baby budget. The cost was

phenomenal. I got an instant headache. I took two Tylenol and went to bed.

<u>2:23 Happy and irritated:</u> Husband called to check up on me, wanted to know if I ate, what I ate, if I was resting, if I left the house.

<u>3:35 Happy and irritated:</u> Mother called to find out same.

<u>4:30 Worried:</u> Is that a twitch or a kick? Is that normal? Can I go the distance? I don't feel high risk! Hmm maybe I am! I should probably go back to bed.

Imagine this is only a few hours in one given day.

- Author

Mental anguish - questions, questions and more questions

For many expectant MoMs pregnancy is one of the happiest periods of their lives. However, for others it can be one of mental anguish with many questions and a lot of thought processes to go through. It is a very emotional time for an expectant MoM as she tries to convince herself that she can go the distance and have a safe delivery of her soon-to-be bundles of joy. Also being labeled as high risk due to the medical complications for both the mom and the fetuses does not make the situation any easier for them to deal with. It is a lot to cope with during this period. The list of questions and concerns is endless, ranging from how they will cope emotionally and financially to what her post pregnancy body may look like!

See the Appendix 2: List of possible questions on the expectant MoM's mind.

Emotional roller coaster

Mood swings are common in most pregnancies. They can be even worse for an expectant MoM with higher levels of hCG (Human chorionic gon-

Concerns and Questions

Top questions of expectant MoMs:
- Can I cope with this?
- Can we handle this financially?
- Will I be on bed rest?
- Will they be premature?
- How will I breast feed them?
- How will I deal with the lack of sleep when they are born?
- What do I need to eat to meet my nutritional needs for all of us?
- How much weight do I need to gain?

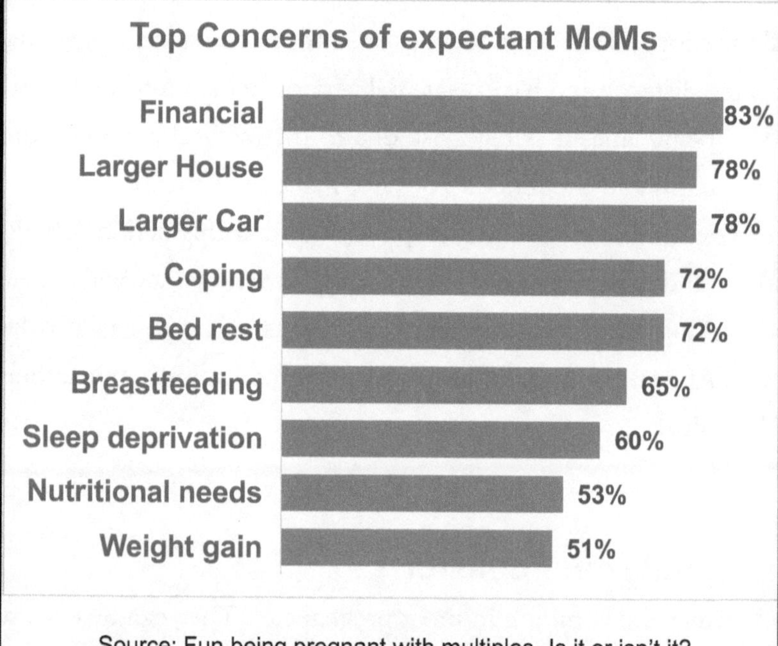

Source: Fun being pregnant with multiples- Is it or isn't it?

adotropin), estrogen and other hormones. She can be fun to be with at one moment and a complete wreck at another. Throughout the pregnancy there will be emotional ups and downs. Some days she may be anxious about the delivery date of her babies and other days she may be over-whelmed by the demands on her body and mind. Many days she may feel that she is not in control of her life. Some women are in a state of denial where they think that all will be well from beginning to end and others may think that everything under the sun will go wrong with them!

> **According to The American Congress of Obstetricians and Gynecologists (ACOG) between 14-23% of all women will struggle with some symptoms of depression in pregnancy**

All this compounds to emotional stress - one of the main triggers of preterm labor. Some expectant MoMs may even develop ante partum depression. It is important for MoMs to control their emotional stress level at this time.

Information Quest

Due to the high risk nature and the complication of her situation, an expectant MoM must be more informed than the average expectant mom about her situation. She must be well read and up to date with what to expect both during the pregnancy and after delivery. She must be very in tune with her body to recognize potentially problematic symptoms. She also needs to formulate and ask all her questions to the best parties and build a network of support. Getting information on her antenatal care may be one of the best ways to ease her worries.

Giving emotional support

My Survey of Present and Prospective Helpers to Mothers of Multiples (MoMs) revealed that many of them had a burning desire to provide emotional support to friends and family members who were expectant parents of multiples (PoMs). Providing this support is easier than you think. When we are under stress, many of us like to have someone to talk to, someone who can relate to our situation or can just be a good listener - a listener that comes without judgment or criticism. Even if you have not had the same experience, some kind, thoughtful words or words of encouragement can make someone feel better about themselves and their situation.

The best ways to show the expectant MoM emotional support are:

- Be genuine, listen, empathize with her
- Allow her to explain her situation, feelings, fears, concerns, thoughts
- Understand what it is like to be pregnant with multiples by reading this book!
- Familiarize yourself with some of the questions she may have (see Appendix 2: List of questions on the mind of the expectant MoM)
- Show that you understand her situation but don't give unsolicited advice
- Find activities that you and the expectant MoM can do together e.g. shopping, dinner, going for a walk, watching a movie
- Encourage her to see beyond the stressful situation and the future that lies ahead with her and her prospective family
- Motivate her to set and achieve short term goals e.g. getting through the week, or a phase, or event, a trimester
- Don't create additional stress. Be helpful, don't burden her with your

problems

- Assure her that you are there for her whenever she needs a listening ear or a shoulder to cry on
- Surprise her with small gifts or gestures to show that you care or that she is in your thoughts and prayers
- Help her find other expectant MoMs or support groups that she may be able to relate to

Know what to say (or not) to an expectant MoM

It does not matter how you found out that your friend or relative is having multiples. There are a host of emotions and questions to follow! There is no end to the amount and type of questions she will get when someone hears that she is pregnant with multiples. They range from her personal feelings to how often she and her partner had sex! And I know you have an array of questions for her too! Some of the questions (I hope) would have been answered in **Chapter 2 - Twins, Triplets - How did that happen!** While others will be answered in the upcoming chapters.

Remember some people hold certain types of information near and dear to them and others will share just about anything. Either way, it is wiser and less embarrassing to both the expectant MoM and yourself if you assume that she is a private person and approach the questioning cautiously.

While you may have a burning desire to know many things about the expectant MoM's situation, it is not about you at this time. It is about her and her babies! Gauge

TIP

She may share that information, but she may just not be comfortable sharing that information with you!

12 things not to say to an expectant MoM

- Better you than me!
- You look very large!
- You look like you are going to have those babies right now!
- I did not know you could get so big!
- Wow, you must have a lot of stretch marks!
- Did you use fertility drugs?
- Were you trying for twins/ triplets?
- Do you think all will survive?
- Do you think that they will have special needs?
- You will definitely need to quit your job!
- Are you making up for lost time?

**Definitely, do not share
pregnancy horror stories!**

her reaction to certain topics; you may be able to slip in some questions that you just need to know or are dying to find out! **The key is to ask meaningful questions.**

Here are a few meaningful questions that you can ask:

- Do you know if they are identical or fraternal?

- What were the reactions of you and your partner?

- Do you feel them moving at the same time?

- What were the reactions of other family members?

- Who knows that you are carrying multiples thus far?

- How are you feeling physically?

- Do you have heartburn, nausea, back pains, pelvic pains, and shortness of breath?

- How do you sleep?

- Do you need pillows or a recliner to help you rest comfortably?

- Are you on any type of movement restrictions? e.g. bed rest
- What are your dietary requirements?
- Do you have any cravings?
- How far along are your nursery preparations?
- What items do you have for your babies thus far?
- What's your view on purchasing gently used items or using hand me downs, borrowed equipment and gear?
- Would you like some music / movies / books / magazines?
- Are you part of any support groups for expectant MoMs?
- Do you have any links with other MoMs/ friends who are MoMs?
- Do you need assistance to attend your doctor's visits e.g. transport, emotional support?
- Who will help you look after your other child/children if/when you are put on bed rest?
- Who is going to look after your other children while you are at the hospital?
- Have you chosen names as yet?
- Do you know their genders?
- What are their present weights?

Researching and Networking

You can be instrumental in helping the PoMs satisfy some of their informational needs. All the information that they will need is not always multiples related and other people may be able to give some advice.

There may be areas you may be able to give input based on your experiences, training or vocation e.g. as a mother, an insurance agent, a nutritionist, a pharmacist, medical practitioner, nurse, midwife, home decorator etc. You can give her some valuable information. Let it be known that you are giving suggestions and they are not orders!

Multiple births are a common phenomenon. Many of us may know someone who has multiples and you may be able to link the PoMs with those families or help her network with more suitable parties. For the tech savvy expectant MoMs there are a lot of online communities, message board forums, chat rooms, blogs and online memberships that can assist her with networking and gaining the supportive responses she needs to keep perspective.

Links to National Multiples Support Groups and websites

Multiples of America	**www.multiplesofamerica.org**
AMBA – Australia	**www.amba.org.au**
Twins Trust	**www.twinstrust.org**
NZMBA - New Zealand	**www.multiples.org.nz**
MBC – Canada	**www.multiplebirthscanada.org**
ICOMBO	**www.icombo.org**

You can assist in the information quest by:

- Investigating the options for financial assistance, statutory entitlements to grants and benefits and income tax deductions, maternity leave entitlement and prevailing legislation
- Researching and locating deals, discounts, coupons and freebies for her
- Searching local newspapers for baby fairs
- Conducting internet searches and recommending websites
- Referring her to blogs, sites, magazines, books
- Getting information on multiples must haves, essentials, non-essentials, product reviews, nursery ideas, second hand and gently used sites and stores
- Joining and encouraging reading and research on Neonatal Intensive Care Unit, special conditions, preterm labor symptoms and other

relevant matters

You can help her increase her network by:

- Encouraging her to join local Mother of Twins (MOTs) and Mothers of Multiples (MoMs) clubs or to start one if there isn't one
- Encouraging her to build a parenting network
- Recommending she join hospital sponsored parenting classes
- Getting recommendations from friends on stores, pediatricians, savings, equipment, techniques etc.
- Linking her with some of your friends or acquaintances that can advise on different areas e.g. decorating, finances, nutrition etc.
- Helping her source or refer her to experts based on her needs e.g. lactation consultants, genetic consultants, twins' organizations, pediatricians etc.

6

Socially
Sneak Peek

What's it like?
- **Getting special attention**
- **Filled with silly questions and stares**
- **Demanding on her marriage**
- **Demanding on her husband**
- **Difficult on her other children**

How can I help?
- **Engage her in fun and relaxing activities**
- **Help her with her other children**
- **Plan and organise a baby shower**

What's it like Socially

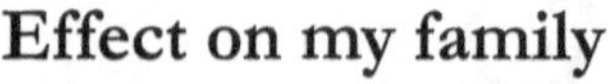

Effect on my family

Emotions were running high during my pregnancy for me, my husband and my other family members as well. Our family does not show much emotion; as a result, everyone went about as if they were fine emotionally. I only knew after the birth of my babies how much stress my family members and my husband were under while I was pregnant. I did not let them know of my fears and my worries and they did likewise. I just wanted to get through my 36 weeks with the least amount of stress and feel as normal as possible and not feel like a caged bird.

My husband was grappling with issues such as how to get an independent, stubborn, workaholic, shopaholic woman pregnant with multiples to take it easy and follow instructions! After the birth of our babies he admitted that fear of preterm labor and my death due to complications, plus all the advice he was getting had him feeling overwhelmed. He did not seem that way to me and he told me I did not seem frustrated. I felt badly for not listening to him during my pregnancy. After all he had my best interest at heart.

My mother was also very scared and did not want to think or speak of the negative possibilities. She lost 20lbs off her small frame while I was pregnant trying to cater to my every need. My sister went beyond the call of duty to ensure that I was comfortable and my babies' clothes, gear and nursery were prepared.

I felt so frustrated being treated like an egg and constantly being

watched, that I decided not to tell the rest of my friends that I was carrying triplets until the third trimester. The real motivation behind this was to be treated like a "normal pregnant woman" and so they were not filled with fear and worry. Also, I did not want to listen to the horror stories they might feel compelled to share and I would still be able to go out and have fun! Less policing!
- Author

Extra attention

One of the advantages of being pregnant with multiples is the pampering and the love and attention you receive from your friends and family members. Even if there are tons of multiples in your family, the novelty of multiples never dies. But while some may relish the additional attention other MoMs may find it overwhelming at times. The extra attention paid may have adverse effects on other family members and children. Some family members may feel that the situation places an additional burden on some of

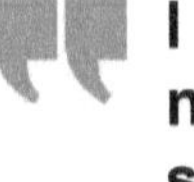

I felt like I was a magnet for stares, horror stories, advice and questions!"
– Expectant MoM

them, as they may have less attention being paid to them or may be given extra duties and chores.

Silly questions and stares

There is no end to the questions that people ask when they know you are carrying multiples. You may need to develop a thick skin, find a sense of humor and keep a few smiles in your pocket to deal with all the questions and attention. It is sometimes a bit shocking the types of questions people will ask and who asks – anyone from the guy on the street corner to the little old lady in your church!

Demanding on her marriage

Being pregnant with multiples places huge demands on both individuals and their marriage. It is also a great source of financial and emotional stress. There are so many demands on the woman that she may focus more on herself and anticipated babies and neglect her husband. Her mood swings and bouts of irritability do not make her or the situation any easier to deal with. Some couples find themselves getting closer during pregnancy, while for others, particularly those with previous marital issues, it may be difficult coping with all the extra demands.

Demanding on her husband

Expectant MoMs are not the only emotional ones at this time. Husbands may feel isolated as all the attention is being placed on the one carrying the babies and not on him. He may feel like a spectator to his own future. Expectant dads must manage their emotions and that of the expectant mom as well. He will be overly concerned about her health and that of the

**Some causes of stress
during pregnancy**

- **Relationship problems**
- **Financial problems**
- **Family or personal history of depression**
- **Previous pregnancy loss**
- **Complications in pregnancy**
- **Exposure to pregnancy horror stories**
- **Unanswered questions**
- **Fear of the unknown - NICU, infant mortality, bed rest, C-section, having children with special needs**
- **Stressful life events**
- **History of abuse or trauma**
- **Work related issues**

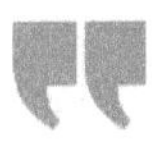

Popular sextuplet and twin mom - Kate Gosselin in May 2009 on her TLC show "Jon & Kate plus 8" stated that MoMs have triple the divorce rate.

Research by MOST (Mothers of SuperTwins) in 2009 showed the US divorce rate for: first marriages was 40%, parents with twins 3.6%, parents with triplets 5%, parents with quadruplets 9.2% and parents with quintuplets/ sextuplets or multiple sets of multiples was 4.2%

"I am glad to know that Kate Gosselin was very wrong!" - Author

babies. He will also be concerned about a host of other things including how this new situation would affect his social life, his pocket and his sex life. There will also be some thinking ahead about what the expectations are of him as a dad and if he'll have to give up his hobbies, be involved in night feedings, perform extra chores etc. The new demands on him may be difficult for him to manage at times; the extra work, chores, errands, doctor's visits and expenses may have him more irritable than usual.

Effects on other children

Having previous children, regardless of their age, adds an additional complication to expecting multiples. Even when energy drained with back aches and morning sickness the expectant MoM cannot forget her other children. They had needs before she was expecting multiples and they surely do not disappear because she is tired or on bed rest or needs to slow down. These children still need to be fed, dressed, played with, spoken to, cooked for, cleaned up after and the list goes on.

Children have emotions too and may also have a hard time dealing with the new restrictions and changes to their lives. Some may even act out in frustration if they do not understand. They need to be remembered, feel part of the family, have fun and socialize even if mom may not always have the energy to help.

How to help with social issues

Engaging her in fun and relaxation

Relaxation is a key element in having a stress-free pregnancy. The expectant MoM has less time than the average expectant mother of a singleton before her delivery date - but she may have more time to be bored. Whether she is on bed rest, total confinement or just resting at home with her feet up, she will need some activities to keep her mind at ease and not occupied with the possibilities of her situation.

Reading is an option, however too much reading about pregnancy related issues may be incredibly stressful after a while. There is a need for some lighter activities for her to participate in while being pregnant; these could be done with a group, family or by herself.

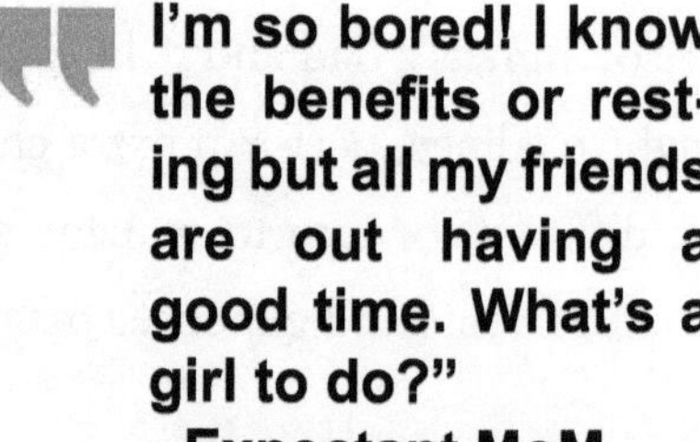

You can help her have some fun and relaxation in her alone time:

- Recommend that she takes up a hobby e.g. photography, craft
- Purchase supplies to support one of her hobbies e.g. art supplies, paint supplies, jigsaw puzzles

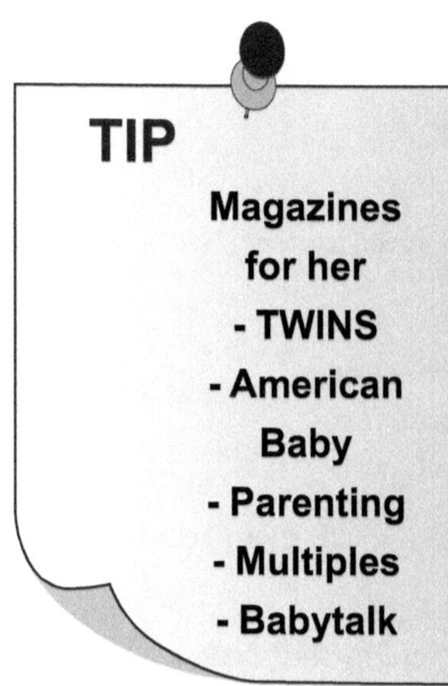

- Buy material for starting and keeping a journal or scrap booking
- Recommend some brain challenging activities e.g. Sudoku, crossword puzzles, online games
- Recommend that she learns a new skill e.g. foreign language, a computer skill, typing
- Recommend some online activities e.g. writing her own blog, joining online groups, creating an online gift registry, keeping family and friends updated using social media, taking an online class
- Purchase books or magazine subscriptions for her on parenting, pregnancy, nursery decorating and other fun stuff
- Purchase movies or a movie subscription
- Give a gift certificate for a spa day and beauty treatment, antenatal massage, manicure or pedicure
- Purchase a gift certificate for photography ante or post natal
- Bring her some comfort food and snacks like ice cream, crackers or fruit
- Recommend some networking activities e.g. taking a parenting class, joining a support group

For fun with the expectant MoM and friends you can:

- Organize a baby moon for her and her significant other
- Suggest some baby names
- Organize or host a baby shower
- Plan a gender reveal activity or event
- Host a spa day e.g. manicures and pedicures for her and her friends

- Take her on a shopping spree
- Purchase fun clothing for her and the babies e.g. multiples themed onesies like two peas in a pod
- Attending Mothers of Multiples sales
- Organize a yard sale to help the MoM clean out her stuff to make room for babies' stuff
- Work on the nursery
- Organize a leisurely lunch with some friends
- Organize brunch with her, friends and family
- Have an evening of non-alcoholic drinks - make them at home or go out
- Invite her and some friends for a girl's evening and some gossip
- Have a movie night with her and some friends either at home or at the cinema
- Host a card tournament
- Be the photographer for some fun photos.

Helping with siblings

Because there are so many things being bought and prepared for the babies, effort must be made to make the other child/children feel special. Close family members, persons with children, persons who like children, persons who may have a child in the same class as the older sibling, teachers and creative persons can all play a role to assist MoM here.

The expectant MoM should also make the effort to help her children become familiar with other grownups and children that he/she may have to deal with while MoM is on bed rest, hospitalized or after the babies are born. You do not want to be seen as a stranger when you are trying to assist MoM with her babies and other children.

To assist the expectant MoM, you can:

- Offer to drop off or pick up siblings from their engagements like soccer practice and gymnastics or from school

- Assist with homework as she may be too tired or not feeling well
- Prepare lunches for the child/ children as Mom may not have the energy or time to do it for him/her
- Arrange to have play dates for the sibling(s)
- Bring over your children or relatives to play with the sibling(s) for a few hours
- Bring toys or a gift for the other sibling(s)
- Engage them in games, movies, activities
- Carry sibling(s) to the mall, for ice cream or to the park to have some fun
- Create activity bags or surprise boxes for the child

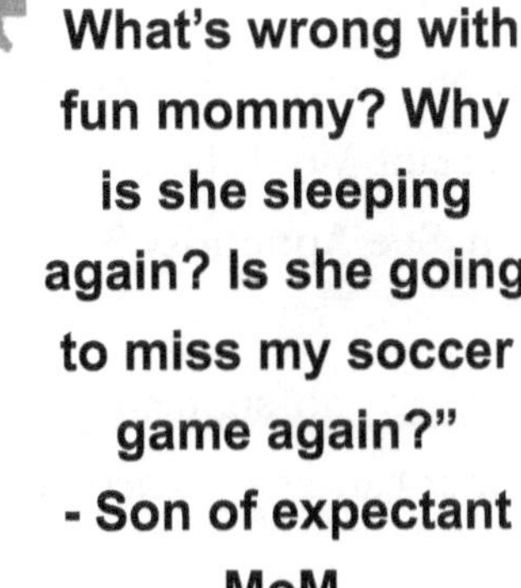

[Activity bag - Activities that can keep a bored toddler occupied and entertained for a while, assembled or made to fit into a bag e.g. for car rides, doctor's office or at home.]

Planning or organizing a baby shower

Baby showers are the greatest and most useful event for MoMs. It can be a simple gathering of a few friends / family members or it can be full scale party with decorations, a theme, a cake, and games etc. However, it is definitely an occasion to have the company of friends and family, get some love and support over some hors d'oeuvres and collect some much needed baby items and advice in the process.

If the expectant MoM isn't aware of this let her know how wise it is to have a baby shower. She will definitely appreciate having a well-planned and organized baby shower. When dealing with a baby shower for an expectant MoM there are a few additional things to take into consideration. **See Appendix 3 - Tips for planning a Shower for Multiples.**

There are no stipulations on the amount of baby showers that one mother can have, whether she could have it for her first child or any

> **Friends, family, food, games and gifts - our baby shower was the best! My friends and family were elated to spend this time with us and it gave them the opportunity to bring us some well-meaning gifts. I was so lucky I got baby stuff to help me through almost the full first year of our babies' lives.**
> **- Expectant PoM**

other etc. If carefully planned, it can relieve the expectant parents of a great financial burden of having to purchase many items. Next time you are invited to a baby shower, be sure to choose a great item from their baby registry or purchase a thoughtful and useful item for them. **See Appendix 4 - Tips for Buying for Twins, Triplets and More.**

To make this event a memorable and successful one for the expectant MoM you can:

- Plan and organize the shower
- Offer your home to host the baby shower
- Make finger foods or provide snacks or drinks
- Help source and organize games for the shower
- Help clean up after the baby shower

- Help pack away gifts after the baby shower
- Write thank you notes to attendees of the shower

7

Physically
Sneak Peek

What's it like?
- **Numerous doctors' visits**
- **Labeled high risk**
- **Risk of preterm labor**
- **Threat of bed rest**
- **A major adjustment**
- **Hormones and exaggerated symptoms**
- **Hungrier than usual**
- **Fluids in and fluids out**
- **Working logistics**
- **Sleeping discomfort**
- **Sex - missing or dreading**
- **Pregnancy brain**

How can I help?
- **Promote healthy eating habits**
- **Be a helpful substitute**
- **Do chores and run errands**

What's it like Medically & Physically

The Flood

One day I came home from a meeting and saw water gushing from the second level of my home. Water was up to my ankles in some places and my knee in others. Things were just floating around my house! How could this be? I instinctively rushed in to investigate and to start moving some items when I saw a vision of my doctor saying, "Triplet mother to be, what do you think you are doing? I said keep bending and lifting to a minimum! Do you ever listen?"

I immediately called my husband and as usual there was no urgency in his voice. I called my mom next. I got a stern warning from her as she shouted, "Do not do anything, I will be there within the hour!" My mom, dad and sister made the one hour drive and came to the rescue. When my husband and my family arrived, I had already managed to move a few things out. My shoes and rugs were sailing! Oh, my beloved shoes! I had to move them! Well, when life gives you lemons…

I decided to make good of the situation and I used that opportunity to start the preliminary preparations on my nursery. After all, I had to remove everything in the room for the mop up and clean-up operations. If this did not happen, I was surely not going to start my preparations any time soon!

Well not listening did have its repercussions. I did not do much more than walk up and down, gasp in horror and move a few very light items. The next day I had a serious back pain and a very strange feeling in my lower abdomen. Was that a twitch? Was that a contraction? Needless to say, I was back at the doctor's office that very afternoon. I had been there for my monthly visit two days previously and the doctor said everything was fine. My doctor's examination and ultrasound indicated that my cervix had started to dilate. He also indicated that I should have a cervical stitch inserted and that the sooner I had it done the better the chances for my babies and me.

What? I was not mentally prepared for a surgery at this time, as minor as it may be. He indicated that we could have the procedure done the day after which was Saturday, Monday or even the next week. I was thinking Monday was a good possibility when my husband blurted out, we will do it tomorrow. What? I looked at him in disbelief. Does my opinion matter anymore? I unwillingly agreed to have the procedure done the Saturday.

- Author

Numerous doctors' visits

From the moment that she finds out that she is carrying multiples, doctor's visits will be longer, more frequent and involved right up until delivery. There will be poking, prodding, questions, testing and ultrasounds at every visit. Genetic testing and fetal heart monitoring are to be expected as well. All these tests are done to determine various important factors including the babies' due date, sex and to monitor fetal growth, possible complications, fetal deformations, the health of the fetus and

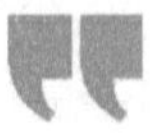

Average # of doctor visits

Normal singleton pregnancy	10-12
My Normal triplet pregnancy	15

possible maternal complications. Needless to say, the cost of prenatal care is much higher than if it were for a singleton.

Labeled high risk

From the day the doctors realize that she is carrying more than one baby the word high risk keeps floating around. After all, the human body was designed to carry one fetus at a time. Multiple births are more likely to run into medical complications than singleton births. However, many expectant MoMs go through their pregnancy smoothly or with only a few complications but the possibility of detrimental effects on her and her babies is a major consideration. She will have to give thought to the possibility of the survival of all her babies and or her babies being born with special needs as the risk of this increases with multiples. Knowing her body, paying attention to warning signs, going to the doctor regularly and having a good relationship with her doctor can help her reduce her risks.

Medical complications
- Maternal complications include spotting, preeclampsia - high blood pressure, gestational diabetes, anemia, placenta previa and abruption placenta.
- Fetal complications include twin to twin transfusion and intrauterine growth restriction.

High risk of preterm labor

In the expectant MoM's case, the risk of pre-term labor and the likelihood of her babies being born prematurely is higher than that of an expectant mother of a singleton. Overcrowding of the uterus alone is sufficient to cause preterm labor but preeclampsia and uterine tumors among other things can also trigger this. Although there are drugs that can be used to slow or stop the onset of labor, extra precaution must be taken at this time. Listening to her doctor and heeding warning signs is vital.

Constant threat of bed rest

Due to the complication of the pregnancy and high preterm labor risk it is almost guaranteed that a period of bed rest will be involved. This can vary from complete confinement at home or in the hospital, resting a few hours with her feet up, or lying down all day. Keeping the weight off her feet and her cervix is particularly important. This can be a challenging period where feeling ill or boredom can be the order of the day. Some expectant MoMs may not be able to do their usual activities like cooking or preparing the babies' room as sitting or standing for long periods is not an option. Resting in a reclined position usually reduces stress and rejuvenates the mind and body.

A major adjustment

On every doctor's visit she hears that she must slow down, get some naps during the day and put her feet up. If she is at work, she may need to sit in a semi reclined position with her feet up for approximately thirty (30) minutes several times of the day. This is difficult for someone who likes to be busy.

If she likes to exercise, caution must be taken. Aerobic exercises and exercises with weights are a definite no. Limited moderate exercise including yoga, walking, swimming and stretching is possible. However, in many cases doctors may advise against any exercise as a precautionary measure to avoid preterm labor.

Hormones and exaggerated symptoms

The average expectant MoM feels more ill than an expectant mother of a singleton during her pregnancy due to the increased hormones and exaggerated symptoms caused by carrying more than one fetus. They experience more morning sickness, nausea, mood swings and bouts of irritability.

She is in what I call "the pressure period" and will definitely be feeling or having some of these symptoms. Some of the discomforts she may feel are shortness of breath due to pressure on her lungs, heartburn due to pressure in her stomach, constipation and hemorrhoids due to pressure on the intestinal tract, back pain due to pressure on her back, pelvic pain from pressure on her pelvis when she stands or the desire to urinate a lot due to pressure on her bladder. This can be a period of great discomfort for many.

Fluids in and fluids out

Doctors usually stress the importance of keeping hydrated during pregnancy. Drinking fluids is highly important as this prevents constipation, helps build cells and additional blood, amniotic fluid and tissue, helps transport nutrients to her babies and remove waste from her system. The sad thing about this is that all that fluid must come back out sooner or later!

Hungrier than usual

Carrying more than one baby is a nutritionally challenging time for an expectant MoM. Generally, many may find themselves in a constant state of hunger, although nausea may affect some people's eating patterns. It is advised that expectant MoMs with poor eating habits see a nutritionist who specializes in high risk pregnancies since early weight gain in her pregnancy has the best and greatest effects in producing babies with healthy birth weights. Healthy birth weights are critical for the future mental and physical health of her babies.

Working logistics

Some MoMs may be able to negotiate time away from work, or a decreased workload while for others it may be difficult. With advances in technology and the increased flexibility of certain jobs, telecommuting may be a feasible option. For financial reasons some expectant MoMs may choose to work for as long as possible before delivery. This may pose a risk to both the expectant MoM and her babies as she needs more rest than in a normal singleton pregnancy to reduce the risk of preterm labor. It is important for her to find out about her eligibility for medical leave and disability insurance for this period, particularly, if she goes on bed rest early or needs extra time off afterward to take care of her babies before she returns to work.

Sleeping discomfort

Getting a good night's sleep may be really difficult many nights for some expectant MoMs. During the pregnancy she will have to alter her sleep positions very often. Sleeping in living room recliners and couches can give her the much needed back support she needs and should be considered as an option. Some nights she

> **My husband told me I had to choose between my six pillows and him in our king-sized bed. Guess which I chose!"**
> **- Expectant MoM**

may end up sleeping in a semi reclined position with a lot of pillows or a body shaped pillow wedged everywhere-- around her knees, stomach, back - until she can get some semblance of comfort. However, it is advised that she lies on her left side to keep the weight off her lungs and to help her organs function better.

Missing or dreading sex

During pregnancy, some women have increased sex drives while for others it may be the total opposite. Being tired and nauseous is a definite mood killer. However not having to worry about contraception can be a definite mood igniter. With the increased hormones and mood swings her husband may never know which mood she is in at any given time. Many men actually confess that they are afraid of hurting the babies and may not be interested in sex at this time. In certain cases, doctors may advise against having sex especially in the last trimester since the contractions of a pleasurable orgasm can induce preterm labor and semen contains prostaglandin, which can stimulate vaginal contractions.

Pregnancy brain

Many expectant MoMs find that their brain is a bit scattered during pregnancy. This may sound silly, but it is amazing the things that an expectant MoM may forget during this stage, ranging from where she put her keys to what she ate for breakfast the day before. This is normal for

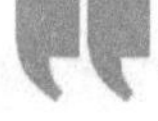

My husband laughed at me every time I whipped out my notebook and pen for my "question and answer sessions" with my OB/GYN"
- Expectant MoM

many during pregnancy so there's no need to be ashamed if it happens, however the expectant MoM may need a note pad, tape recorder or some kind of extra help to remember all the information given to her by her doctor.

My symptoms

I definitely did not feel high risk at all! I did not have morning sickness. I had slight nausea that seemed to kick in at three every afternoon. I slept with Tums under my pillow and never left home without it. Why call it morning sickness if it can happen any time of day?

I had a constant dull migraine in the first trimester, intermittent back pains and mild pelvic pain in the last trimester. Yet I felt like a Spartan! There I was nervously awaiting all these really bad symptoms that I read about but they never came. I would watch expectant mothers of singletons moan, groan and complain at my doctor's office and I would just smile. Feeling my munchkins move was the most thrilling yet strange experience ever. I would get some punches to my stomach from baby #1, some back strokes in the middle of my belly from baby #2 and some kicks to my bladder from baby #3. My babies were all nocturnal because they did not act up during the day. They started at 10pm and gave the last movements just before it was time to go to work!

I was a picky eater before I was pregnant but that changed. I ate without guilt! My husband used to cook the tastiest, nutritious meals I ever had. However, after my hearty meals I would feel as if my stomach was pushed up to under my neck and my food and babies were fighting for space!

For a few months one of my babies was resting on my bladder. If

I drank one glass of water, I would go to the bathroom three times within the hour after this! Night time was even worse. I would manage to sleep for half an hour before I had to roll out of bed to use the bathroom. I had to change bedrooms to be near enough to the bathroom to ensure I had no accidents! My husband jokingly mentioned that I might need to use mattress covers before our babies had to use them!
- Author

How to help physically

Promote healthy eating habits

Amidst the uncertainties involved in getting her babies to full term, there are two things the expectant MoM can control to give her babies a fighting chance of being healthy: #1 what and how much she eats and #2 how much rest she gets!

Here is some simple, but important information about her dietary requirements:

The expectant MoM needs to:

- Eat often - 3 meals and 2-3 snacks per day, every 3-4 hours if expecting twins and 2-3 hours if expecting triplets and quadruplets
- Ingest additional calcium, folic acid, protein, iron and all other nutrients.
- Eat lean proteins, healthy fats and carbohydrate rich foods
- Intake an additional 300 calories per day per baby
- Keep hydrated

A great informational source for nutritious meals and snacks is When expecting – Twins, Triplets or Quads by Dr. Barbara Luke and Tamara Oberlin. This book has 75 original recipes and 120 nutritious menu suggestions for meals and snacks organized by trimester and broken down into its nutritional content. The expectant MoM, her family or friends can use this as a guide.

To help the expectant MoM in her nutrition battles:

- Bring comfort food like premium ice cream or a basket of nutritious goodies
- Order healthy foods from fast food restaurants
- Bring her lots of fluids to drink like water, fruit juice, milk and sparkling water
- Bring her tummy soothing snacks like crackers, lemons, candied ginger, peppermint tea
- Bring nutritious snacks like nuts, dried fruit, cereals, granola bars
- Deliver fresh or frozen food
- Cook or purchase nutritious food for the expectant MoM
- Cook and freeze foods for the post delivery period
- Deliver meats, multigrain breads and cereals, frozen or low sodium canned vegetables, fruits

Be a helpful substitute

Fun helping out

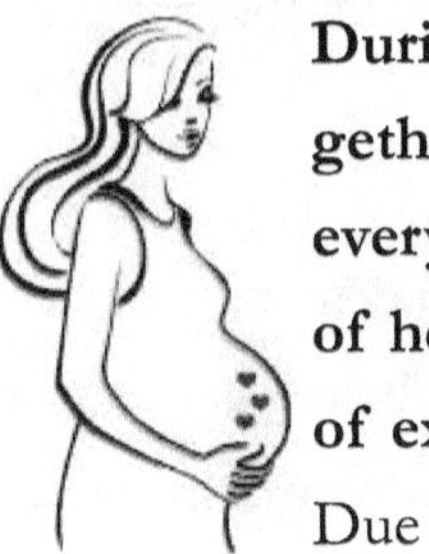

During my sister's pregnancy, we really had fun together. Baby shopping, doctor visits, movies - we made everything into an outing to relieve her of the pressure of her having to do them herself or by herself! – Sister of expectant MoM

Due to the frequency of doctors' visits for the expectant

MoM, dads may not always be available to attend all the doctor's appointments and other engagements. In that case, the expectant MoM may need someone to accompany her to her doctor's appointment or be there for moral support. There may also be other engagements that Dad may not be able to or may be less enthusiastic to attend. In some cases, there may be engagements where it may be more enjoyable or less daunting to have either her sister, mother, or close friend attend instead of her husband. Here is a chance for you to fill in! You can be instrumental in getting her to her engagement or attending it with her. Remember, the aim is not to replace her husband or diminish his role, but to make the expectant MoM happy.

Some opportunities for you to help includes:

- Attending doctor's visits with pen and notepad and be attentive
- Touring of the NICU
- Attending special parenting classes
- Baby shopping
- Internet shopping
- Help in setting up the baby registry
- Seeking out sales - garage sales, consignment stores, online sales

Do chores and run errands

For the expectant MoM, getting rest is especially important, and it increases exponentially as the pregnancy progresses. She has to slow down and be extremely careful due to the high risk nature of the pregnancy and the high risk of preterm labor.

The expectant MoM should list the things that need to take place to keep her household running to aid in the division of labor. Between her husband, her family members or friends she can get many of her things done if they are itemized. This makes it easy for others to identify what they can do to help and gives her more time to relax, eat, rest, read and keep her feet up.

You can help the expectant MoM with the following:

- Itemize, identify and co-ordinate the help she needs during bed rest or after the babies are born
- Assist with the grocery shopping
- Assist with household chores e.g. put a load of laundry in the washer, a load of dishes in the dishwasher, fold some clothes while you chat
- Recommend or source household help or a maid service
- Run for supplies that she may need
- Drop off a bag of groceries for her and her family
- Check in when at the mall, supermarket or pharmacy - you may be able to pick up a few items for her
- Pay bills for her, if she does not pay them online

8

Physical Appearance
Sneak Peek

What's it like?
- **Weight gain**
- **Clothing dilemma**
- **Pregnancy glow**
- **Stretch marks**

How can I help?
- **Assist with maternity shopping**
- **Pamper her**

What's it like- Physical Appearance

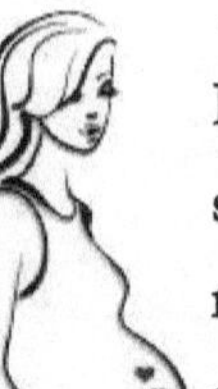

The glow

I don't consider myself to be vain but I was very conscious of my physical appearance while I was pregnant. I went shopping for some trendy pants, leggings and some figure flattering tops. I really dislike seeing pregnant women looking frumpy and unkempt. There are too many available options for maternity clothes!

During the first trimester, I had a case of brittle nails and breaking hair but that changed tremendously during the next two trimesters. I never looked so radiant. I was a hot, very pregnant momma! I got a short trendy hair style to make it easier to manage. When I looked good, I felt better mentally. It made it easier to say, "Suck it up Sharlene! Your babies are feeding off your energy!"

One issue that I really couldn't shake off was the first appearance of stretch marks. It took me months to get over it. I tried **Palmers Cocoa butter** and **Bio Oil** but neither of them worked for me. Sometime in the third trimester I accepted that it was a small price to pay to deliver three healthy babies.

My body was more or less the same size but my belly was huge! Turning heads with over 50lbs of belly and I couldn't even see my toes! What an ego booster! Even on the days that I felt under the weather I would dress up and appear to be feeling well! Even when I was on bed rest at the hospital, I carried my hair dryer, curling iron and nail polish and made sure I looked and felt good! There is an upside to being pregnant, carrying around a large belly and looking like you are a few months more advanced than you really are! People are usually always willing to help! People offer you their space in the line. Heck you get to go to the front of the line. They offer to push your trolley and unpack your groceries. Oh yes, and they bring you lots of gifts and yummy treats! Let them know that you are carrying multiples - Ah! They treat you like a queen! The downside is that they also treat you like a cracked egg.

- Author

Weight gain

The weight gain for an expectant MoM is greater than that of an average expectant mom. She will definitely get more stares and comments due to her size or her waddling around. At six months an expectant mother of twins

Average weight gain
Singleton | 25-35lbs
Twins | 37-54lbs
Triplets | 50-60lbs

marchofdimes.org

looks like she is eight months pregnant and an expectant mother of triplets looks full term! The extra weight also can make her tired easily and quickly. A woman carrying twins at 30 weeks is carrying the same weight as a singleton mom at full term. Just when you think that she can't get any larger she does!

A clothing dilemma

Finding comfortable, trendy clothing for an expectant MoM is quite a task. For starters, she will gain weight quickly and she will need to do maternity shopping earlier and quite of-

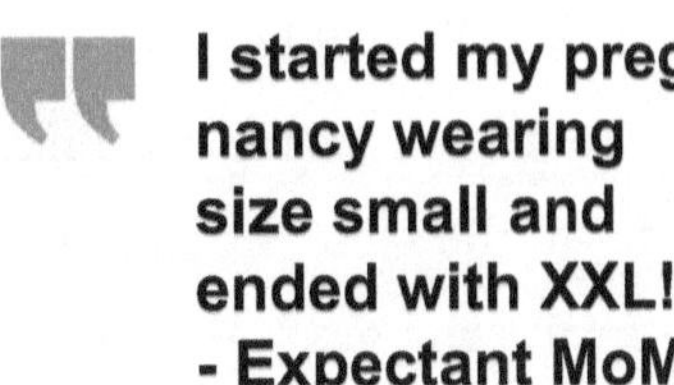

ten. Although weight gain in the early trimesters is beneficial to the babies, it will be quite frustrating to open the closet and find that her clothes don't fit or that she purchased shoes or clothing and in a matter of weeks they no longer fit.

There are so many options these days for maternity clothes but she will have to make some thoughtful choices. She will definitely need the clothes sooner, grow out of them faster and be in them longer after birth than a singleton mom! Gone are the days where a pregnant woman hides in her husband's shirts and sweatpants. Stylish, practical, good fitting, and high-quality maternity clothing are available.

Pregnancy glow

Maintenance of hair, nails and skin can be fun for some expectant MoMs. Some are lucky to grow longer hair and stronger nails while others are unfortunate to develop brittle nails and breaking hair. Also many pregnant women develop that extra radiance or pregnancy glow, caused by an increase in blood flowing close to the skin's surface. However, it can be an overwhelming nightmare for others as they may develop skin blemishes, tight and itchy skin, acne, skin discoloration or sensitivity to skin care products and the sun.

Stretch marks

Some women may develop issues with her new pregnancy figure as she wonders how she looks to her husband, how she will look post pregnancy and how she will lose her pregnancy weight. Other pregnant women worry about stretch marks, a natural and sometimes inescapable consequence of the skin stretching for the growing babies. However, these are some of the many things that she will have to accept.

How to help her physical appearance

Maternity shopping

Shopping when expecting multiples can be quite a challenge. Her list of things to buy may also include some non-traditional items that may now seem to be a maternity necessity. A good example is a recliner or glider to rest and relax or books and magazines to pass those boring days on bed rest. The expectant MoM may be less than enthusiastic to shop by herself as weight gain will cause her to tire easily or experience pain in her feet. She may also need an extra pair of eyes or an opinion to help her decide on what to purchase. Shopping for her new shape and size can be overwhelming and tiring.

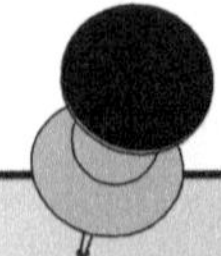

TIP

Gift ideas for expect- ant MoM

- Shoes - slip on, flats, sandals, flat sole boots, sneakers
- Belly support
- Maternity / nursing bra
- Body / maternity pillow
  Maternity clothes
- Antenatal massage
- Gift certificate for a spa
- Recliner
- Favorite movies / movie sub- scription
- Books (pregnancy and baby)
- Magazines or subscription
- Basket of goodies
- Accessories - jewelry, scarves
- Photo album
- Camera
- Hair and skin products

Some ways to assist her in maternity gear and wear:

- Help her shop or purchase or lend her a comfortable recliner/glider
- Help her purchase some figure flattering maternity wear
- Lend or pass along some of your maternity wear
- Surprise her with or accompany her to purchase accessories to go with her new wardrobe
- Suggest or go with her to consignment or thrift stores to purchase gently used maternity clothing or other items
- Shoe shop with her
- Purchase her favorite movies, music, books or magazines

Pampering

While the expectant MoM is trying anxiously to carry her babies to term, she may forget to take care of herself and there may also be days during her pregnancy where she may not feel her best. Both mommy and babies need to be taken care of. You can give her the extra encouragement and a reminder to take time to take care of herself as well.

Some ways to give her the extra encouragement:

- Bring her skin soothing solutions and moisturizers
- Give a skin care gift basket with pregnancy safe hair care and skin care products
- Refer her to a dermatologist for her skin care issues
- Research with her the best over the counter skin and hair care solutions
- Give a gift certificate for a spa day, beauty treatment, antenatal massage, manicure or pedicure
- Give a gift certificate to the hairdresser
- Give her a manicure or pedicure or paint her nails in some cheerful colors

9

Financially
Sneak Peek

What's it like
- **More expensive than a singleton**
- **Expenses, expenses and more expenses**
- **Brings on cost consciousness**

How can I help?
- **Kick start the baby shopping**
- **Give a financial contribution**
- **Source cost savings**

What's it like Financially

How much is this going to cost us?

Being accustomed to living in a dual income home, I started to worry about the financial impact of my pregnancy, more than my husband. While he was worried about my health, I was worried about my spending power. Giving up my income to go on bed rest and then child birth was a painful thought. I love to spend money. Frugally of course! Immediately my husband began to look at investments, working longer hours and decreasing expenses as ways to increase our income both in the short term and in the long term.

I missed him while he was working his new longer hours but I also saw the expenses racking up. It started with the expenses of the doctor's visits, then the additional tests to be done, then it was the additional maternity clothes that I quickly out grew, the extra supplements to ensure our babies were born healthy, the additional food stuff since I ate all day, and the list continued.

The first time cost of multiples is mind boggling! One afternoon I constructed my budget for the upcoming expenses for diapers, formula, baby clothes and gear, the essentials and some "nice to have items"; I felt overwhelmed by the expenses, got depressed and went to bed. I did not speak about it for about a week; after this I was actually able to verbalize the cost. I felt poor! We were in a fairly good financial position pre pregnancy but this was definitely going to make us broke, if we did not act wisely!

I glimpsed a report that indicated that a middle-income family with a child born in 2011 can expect to spend about a quarter of a million dollars for food, shelter, and other necessities (excluding college) to raise that child over the next 17 years. And that was for one child! I had sleepless nights wondering how we were going to cover our future expenses.

- Author

Filled with expenses, expenses and more expenses!

My **Survey of Mothers of Multiples (MoMs)** revealed that "How having and raising multiples will affect them financially," was a major concern while they were pregnant.

The cost of additional maternity clothes, supplements and food stuff all add up. And that's only the cost of the pregnancy! Budgeting for wipes, milk, baby clothes and gear, the essentials and the nice to haves, childcare, and possibly a larger house and car, has to be done before these expenses start rolling in. Another important consideration is the financial impact of being on bed rest or extended leave and the possibility of having newborns with special needs and an extended stay at the hospital.

More expensive than carrying a singleton

Cost of raising a child born in 2012 to the age of seventeen (college not included):

    $173,490 - lower income families

    $241,080 - average income families

    $399,780 - higher income families

                      USDA News

Needless to say, carrying multiples is more expensive than carrying a singleton. Although the prenatal visits cost may be the same, the cost of prenatal care is higher due to the more frequent visits to the doctor and the additional tests to get done. Also, physicians charge more for the delivery of multiples than singletons due to the complexity of the delivery.

Brings on cost consciousness

Every time you think of your future bundles of joy, you see dollar signs. Also, every time you think of purchasing something, you automatically do the multiplication like a reflex, even if you know that everything is not needed in multiples! Buying in bulk, looking for sales, clipping coupons, discounts and freebies begin to look much more attractive when you know you are carrying more than just one baby. Thrift stores and consignment shops are a good source of bargains. A MoM may also be the beneficiary of generous gifts from friend and family.

> I was never one to want secondhand items, hand me downs or pass-alongs. I love the new clothes smell! I love to see the items in their new boxes and plastic! But after I saw how quickly my babies grew out of stuff and got fed up with stuff I was very happy to accept them. Raising babies ain't cheap!"
> - Expectant MoM

How to help financially

Kick start the baby shopping

There is definitely a lot of shopping to be done for the preparation for multiples. Some expectant MoMs may have a baby registry which will

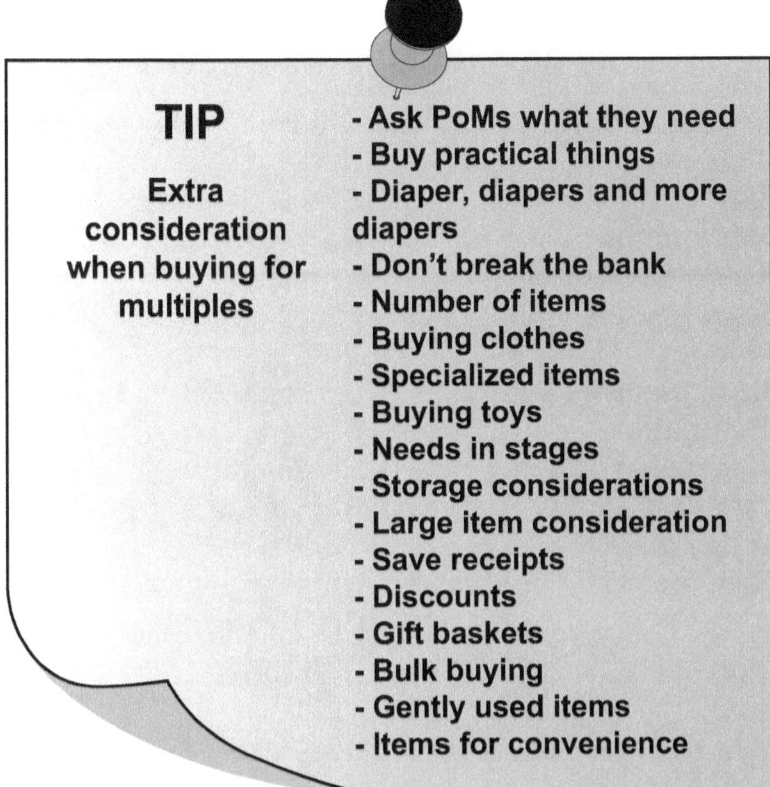

make it much easier for her friends and family to know what to purchase for her. Basically she has already determined what she wants and you just have to choose what you would like to get her.

If she does not have a baby registry you will have to rack your brain to decide on the best gifts to get her. Not to add any pressure, but there is an additional amount of consideration that you need to give purchasing for the expectant MoM and her multiples. **See Appendix 4 - Tips on buying for Twins, Triplets and More.**

To help the expectant MoM you can:

- Help offset some of the new recurring expenses by purchasing diapers, wipes, or formula
- Purchase items from her baby registry

Top 25 gifts for an expectant MoM

- Diapers and wipes
- Onesies
- Bibs
- Bottle props
- Hands free bottles
- Bouncy seats
- Swings
- Plush blankets
- Play mats
- Chic diaper bag
- Car seats
- Boppy pillow
- White board

- Gift baskets with essentals
- Sleepers/footed pajamas
- Receiving blankets
- Strollers
- Fitted crib sheets
- Baby monitor
- Large diaper bag
- Camera
- Photo album
- Baby sling or front carrier
- Nursing pillow
- Daily schedule book

- Assist her in purchasing items off her list of essentials
- Purchase an item from either the top 25 gifts or after reading **Appendix 4: Tips for buying for Twins, Triplets and More.**
- Take her shopping to give some advice if you have any experience in this area
- With her input, purchase one of the big ticket items on the MoM's list
- Enlist friends or family members to purchase one of the big ticket items e.g. strollers, cribs, playpens
- Assemble gift baskets or hampers for her e.g. diapering essentials, feeding essentials, first aid kit, laundry essentials for baby.

Give a financial contribution

Giving financial contributions may be a contentious gift for some and perfectly within the capabilities of others. Relatives, the time constrained or the financially capable may feel comfortable giving a financial contribution toward the newborn babies. You can decide whether it will be a one time, a monthly or an annual contribution. When all is said and done it will be appreciated. If you have wishes in terms of what you want them to do with the money or how it should be used you can indicate this. You can start a college fund or a mutual fund for the children or give good old fashioned cash or a check towards the baby expenses to be incurred by the parents.

On another note, not everyone is willing to accept a financial contribution. It may be more easily accepted if you attach a thoughtful card or some inspirational words or give a gift certificate towards purchasing items for the baby or the household.

Some ideas for financial support are:

- Set up a mutual fund account or college fund for the children
- Make a monthly or annual financial contribution toward the children
- Pay for necessary services or contribute toward e.g. babysitting, house cleaning
- Give gift certificates for purchasing baby clothes and gear
- Gift certificate for Wal-Mart/ Target/ local grocery store / Super-store

Source cost savings

Raising multiples will obviously be more expensive than raising a singleton, however it does not have to be twice and three times the cost. You can help the PoMs by identifying some thrifty ways of saving money.

Loans, hand me downs, pass-alongs - There are a lot of items that may be 'nice to have' for a singleton but is a necessity for multiples e.g. bouncy chairs, play yards, bottle props. Loans, hand me downs, pass alongs also go a long way. They are good for the environment, are an excellent source of cost savings and a great way for MoM to cover her list of necessities and nice to haves. Children wear the clothes and use the toys and equipment for such a short time you can rotate toys and equipment among friends.

Secondhand options - Local PoMs club biannual sales, kids' consignment stores, online shops, garage sales, and thrift stores are all feasible options for gently used baby clothes, toys and equipment. These are sometimes good options when you need multiples of an item or a variety of items without breaking the bank.

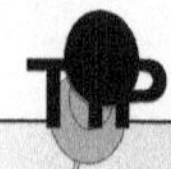

One must ensure the items are in good working order, free from stains and odors, have all their snaps, zippers and parts and should not be recalled or past their expiry date.

Bulk buying – Some items are used more frequently and best purchased in bulk e.g. formula, diapers, wipes, baby food. Bulk buying meats and household necessities like toilet paper, detergent and foodstuff can create great cost savings and save MoM from making several trips to the supermarket after her delivery, because she definitely will not have the time or energy to do this.

Multiple birth programs - Many companies have multiple birth programs and once your case is approved you are granted access to coupons, discounts and freebies. In some cases, you may get discounts when purchasing for multiples only if you ask. It does not hurt to ask.

TIP

One of the most comprehensive and up-to-date lists of freebies and discounts offered to MOMs is available at the Raising Multiples web site.

Ways to help her save includes:

- Loan or pass along baby clothing, gear and toys that are in good condition
- Locate MoM sales, kids' consignment stores etc. or carry MoM or purchase some items for her
- Help her source free items, multiples and rewards programs, coupons and discounts for formula, diapers and toy companies
- Swapping coupons with her on items she will use
- Cut out or create a coupon book on items for the babies e.g. diapers, wipes and baby food
- Encourage her to join a warehouse club for bulk buying
- Offer to baby sit when the babies are born as childcare is expensive
- Check out Raising Multiples (https://www.raisingmultiples.org) for discounts, freebies and coupons for MoMs

10

Bed Rest
Sneak Peek

What's it like?
- **My bed rest story**

How to help?
- **Know what to say (or not) to the expectant MoM**
- **Do chores and run errands**
- **Give emotional support**
- **Pamper her**
- **Kick start the baby shopping**
- **Promote healthy eating habits**
- **Help her with her other children**
- **Engage her in fun and relaxing activities**
- **Plan and organise as the due date comes near**

What's it like - Bed rest

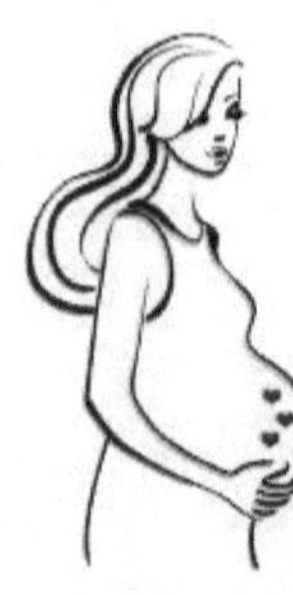

My bed rest story

I woke up feeling exceptionally energetic. Despite my husband's recommendation to head to the OB/GYN's office and return home immediately afterward, I made my list of things to do after my OB/GYN visit. Hmmmm. Let's see.

- Head to the baby store and look at a few 'nice to haves' on my list
- Stock up on the rest of my groceries
- Meet with my sister to unwillingly put the finishing touches on my baby shower that was on Saturday
- and anything else that the day permits.

OB/GYN - Everything looks fine; you are almost at 32 weeks so I think we will see you here tomorrow morning at 8 o'clock

Me - What? You're kidding right. You just said everything was fine

OB/GYN - Everything is fine and we would like to keep it that way! We will admit you for bed rest and for monitoring tomorrow and we can schedule you for delivery next week or the week after

Me - But I feel fine and I can rest at home

OB/GYN - I know, but WE will feel much more comfortable with you here!

This was my conversation with my **OB/GYN** at 32 weeks into my pregnancy. It was a relatively unproblematic one. Nothing out of the ordinary, very little complaints so I was active most of the time. Being independent, I relished the ability to do things myself at my own time without having to ask anyone else to do them. Yes,

I had to waddle around a bit but I got it done all the same!

I was not happy by this. A ton of thoughts popped into my head:

Is he crazy?

Don't they know I still have things to do?

We discussed bed rest as a necessity only if something was wrong

Was something wrong?

So why can't I rest in my own bed?

Had they found out about my inability to sit still for more than five minutes?

I was feeling great. No pains. No discomfort.

This has to be a conspiracy.

He managed to give me two days to organize myself. Two days? I thought I had at least another four weeks. I had things to do, people to see and the list went on.

Sigh! So, the woman who liked to do it all was lying in the hospital, bored and with things that I thought were important to do still to be done! Think quickly, what do I have? A note pad and my mobile phone. Think again! I had my list of contacts – my window to the world. I hated delegating but I had no choice.

I never considered myself as having a lot of friends and I usually tried to do everything myself, but it was amazing how many people were willing to take a few minutes out of their schedule to assist me. I had not considered that in any of my planning sessions during my pregnancy. I did not even have to ask; people were willing to help. I just needed to make sense of it and accept it!

My friends and family made bed rest as enjoyable and comfortable as possible. I enjoyed the attention. As they visited or called, they would ask what I needed or would bring or do what they thought was needed.

I must say it was difficult to move over and let someone else take over. But in retrospect it was the only way to ensure that I gave birth to healthy babies given the high risks involved.

Thank you to all my helpers. Your assistance has been truly appreciated and continues to be.

- Author

Help During Bed Rest

A period of bed rest during her pregnancy is almost guaranteed! For some it can be for as little as a week and for others it could be for the duration of the pregnancy. It can also vary from resting a few hours with her feet up to lying down all day, complete confinement at home or monitoring at the hospital.

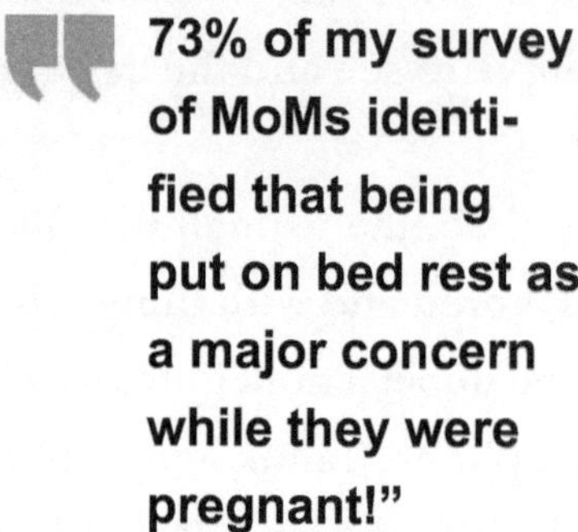

It can be a very emotional and physically uncomfortable period for many MoMs. Countless expectant MoMs have their preparations and plans cut short by unexpectedly early bed rest. They may definitely need someone to finish their plans like shopping and preparing the nursery or packing for the hospital. Also, when she goes to deliver her babies, her household still has to run and be ready for when she returns with her bundles of joy.

Meaningful questions for the expectant MoM on bed rest

- How are you feeling physically?
- Any heartburn, nausea, back pain, pelvic pain, or shortness of breath?
- What type of bed rest are you on?
- Do you need any pillows to help you rest comfortably?
- What are your dietary requirements?
- Would you like some music / movies / books / magazines / newspapers?
- Do you have any one to look after your other children?
- Do you need help paying your bills or are they being paid online or via another arrangement?
- Do you have any chores that you would like done?
- Is the nursery prepared or all the baby essentials purchased?
- Are your hospital bags packed?

To help the expectant MoM on bed rest

- Emotional support
- Run errands e.g. grocery shopping
- Support her food cravings and supplementation
- Cook or bring nutritious meals
- Help with household chores
- Set up the nursery
- Prepare the house for babies' arrival e.g. cleaning, finishing touches on the nursery
- Take care of other children e.g. driving them to obligations
- Locate garage sales, consignment shops and other bargains
- Explore gently used items and lending items
- Purchase items for her hospital bag and for the babies

- Baby shopping
- Bring her favorite movies / music / magazines / books
- Bring books/ magazines on parenting of multiples e.g. - twinsmagazine.com
- Recommend websites and support groups that she can join
- Recommend online pregnancy message boards
- Link her with other MoMs that you may know
- Investigate options for financial assistance
- Take pictures and measure MoM's belly
- Give baby name suggestions
- Pamper her e.g. styling hair, polishing fingernails and toenails

11

Giving Birth

Sneak Peek

What's it like?
- **Contractions or not**
- **Delivery Options**
- **Pain Management**
- **Full House**

How can I help?
- **Help with preparations before babies arrive**
- **Assistance while MoM is hospitalized**
- **Assistance during those first few weeks**

What's it like giving birth to all those babies

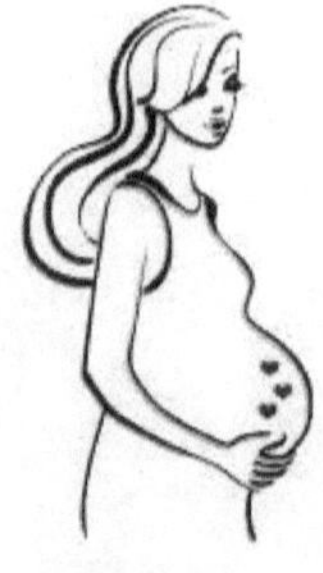

Pregnancy finale

After some weeks of bed rest and months of monitoring every pain and twitch - which thankfully turned out to be a false alarm in every case - I had a long shower while coming to terms with today being "the day."

They wheeled me into the examination room. On my way down the corridor I saw a lot of people watching and waving and wishing me all the best. I watched them dazed. Today was the day - 36 weeks, 5 days, 60 lbs heavier - I was going to give birth to my babies. As I entered the examination room, I saw my husband among the various people who were there. There were more than 40 persons in that examination room. They introduced themselves and tried to lighten the mood although they were all going to be up to some serious business. It was overwhelming at first but soon after they all disappeared in my mind.

My husband held my hand as I got the local anesthetic and then the epidural. I wanted to be fully conscious when my babies arrived. I also had a very close friend who was also a doctor in the examination room. He was there for moral support for us both! My husband did his best to calm my nerves, while our friend tried to keep him calm.

My doctors were very friendly and my main **OB/GYN** was funny too. As he did the procedure, he explained what was going on behind the screen that was obscuring my vision. I could feel a lot of pulling and tugging but no pain. It was the strangest feeling ever. I felt him reaching far inside up under my stomach like he was stuffing a Thanksgiving turkey! I was anxious to meet my babies! I hoped and prayed that they would all be fine, they would all be alive, well, healthy and of good birth weight so they would not have to remain in the neo natal intensive care unit. I did not even remember to pray that I would make it through the surgery.

The first 25 minutes seemed long. My blood pressure kept rising as I anxiously awaited the cry of my first child. "Oh God. Let my baby cry. I've been praying for today for weeks. I was praying to be able to keep them safely inside of me until 36 weeks and I did it. One more step and we are there," I thought anxiously.

I looked at my husband; he was holding my hand and rubbing my head. He was also looking on at the procedure in his usual calm manner. He is a veterinarian and had performed several C-sections in his career but never had he seen a human C-section up close and never on someone he loved.

I looked up at him and saw his facial expression change; before I could try to ascertain what the look meant, I heard my daughter cry. I was never so happy in my life.
"Would you like to hold your daughter?" the doctor asked.
"No thanks, you just keep going. I need to hear them all cry!" I blurted out but I caught a quick glimpse. She was so beautiful. And then after the longest minute of my life I heard another cry. It was my second daughter. She was so tiny and beautiful too. As I tried to lean over to see them both I heard a scream, louder and

more demanding than the first two. That was my son. He was smaller than the first two but as loud as the first two combined! The operating room was like an assembly line; everyone had their tasks and they were all busy and it did not seem chaotic! Well-orchestrated! They wrapped and brought my three bundles of joy, my three miracles. My two daughters got cozy and lay on my chest but my son immediately began looking to suckle. The nurses and the doctors had a hearty laugh. He was quite demanding, while the other two were very quiet. I was so emotional and they were so comfortable. The moment was surreal. The day my babies said hello to the world! February 16th, 2012: Kalicia 1:56pm, Kaylene 1:57pm and Kevin Jr. 1:58pm.

- Author

Contractions or not?

Anxiety is heightened and while some are happy to have their babies as soon as possible, there are others praying for another day to ensure the proper development of their babies. It is important that she knows how to identify when labor has begun. Many women mistake Braxton Hicks contractions with true labor contractions. Braxton Hicks contractions are felt throughout pregnancy. They are irregular and disappear with rest and hydration. True labor contractions are regular and last 30-60 seconds. It is important to differentiate between them as true labor means she has to get to the hospital immediately, as delivering multiples can be complicated. She must be extra vigilant and prepared.

Delivery options

The OB/GYN and the expectant MoM would have discussed her delivery options before her delivery date during her many prenatal visits. Most triplets and all quadruplets are delivered by cesarean section and this is scheduled in advance. All efforts are made not to have her go into labor at all. Vaginal delivery of twins may be safe in circumstances, where the lowest infant is in the head-first position. This accounts for approximately a quarter of twin births. The rest are delivered via C-section. In some cases, the first may be born vaginally, but complications like excessive bleeding, umbilical cord problems or lowered fetal heart rate may cause a C-section to follow. Appropriate anesthesia and neonatal support are critical, whether delivery is performed vaginally or requires cesarean section.

Pain management

Before the date of delivery, she should familiarize herself with the pain management options, their pros and their cons. Relaxation techniques and breathing exercises can assist with labor pains, however analgesics are needed in most cases.

(Analgesics - lessens but does not eliminate pain e.g. morphine, Demerol Anesthesia - produces numbness with or without loss of consciousness e.g. epidural block, local anesthesia, general anesthesia)

Full house

One thing that is guaranteed at the delivery of multiples is the additional people in the operating room. Delivery of multiples requires planning by the entire medical team and availability of full intensive-care support following birth. This may include the obstetrician, a team of neonatologists (one or more for each baby), pediatric nurses, and any other doctors and nurses who will assist with the surgery. In many cases it is a less than private affair. Some hospitals allow the father in the room - hopefully, he does not get queasy at the sight of blood. There may even be a camera crew from the media or the hospital, people looking in from behind the huge window or trainee nurses and doctors as well. If she is awake during her surgery it can be very overwhelming!

Help as the due date comes close

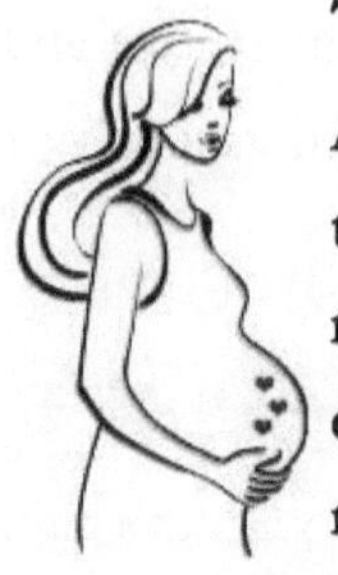

To plan or not to plan!

As much as I am a compulsive planner, I was a little superstitious and reluctant to start preparing my nursery. I definitely needed an extra push to finish it on time. Then although feeling fine I was put on bed rest. My helpers had to rally and finish the job!
- Author

Preparing for the arrival of multiples can be overwhelming, yet exciting. There are moments of great anxiety and anticipation. There is a lot to do, less than the average 40 weeks of pregnancy to do it and she has a lot of physical constraints. The expectant MoM will need more help than the average expectant mom when preparing for her baby as there are some additional considerations in her case.

Here are a few:

- **Shorter prep time -** She needs to start nursery preparations earlier, preferably in the second trimester when she is not as large, not in as much discomfort, on bed rest or on activity restriction. She can't count on the last two months for preparation.

- **Pregnancy brain –** She may forget a lot of stuff she needs to do so getting it done early is the best precaution.

- **Room vs. rooms / crib vs. cribs -** She must determine how she will set up to accommodate more than one baby and the items, equipment and clothing they need.

- **Baby stations -** These are separate areas in the house, set up to accommodate baby feeding and cleaning. It is helpful especially when there is more than one baby as you can save on trips up and down the stairs and it's easier to function while you are cooking, eating or doing laundry etc.

- **Balancing time** - Dealing with more than one baby and running the household, looking after children, doing chores, cooking etc.
- **Baby proofing -** To accommodate more than one as it is difficult to keep your eyes on more than one baby at a time.
- **Larger car** - To fit babies, the rest of the family and her gear as well.
- **Cost and practicality** of things like how much of certain items to buy such as cloth or disposable diapers, new or gently used items or to breastfeed or use formula feeding.
- **Matching / coordinated outfits** or not
- **Larger house or home modification** - Repurposing furniture or rooms may be necessary e.g. conversion of a dining room or living room to accommodate a baby station with changing gear, bouncy chairs, swings, play mats, pack and plays.
- **Décor** - The theme, the color, the characters and the design can vary based on the mix of genders of the multiples.

Help with preparation before delivery of babies

- Assist in setting up the nursery from painting to allocating space and decorating
- Give décor tips for nursery and other areas in the house to prep for babies' arrival
- Set up stations in different areas of the house to decrease the number of trips to get things done
- Create diaper changing baskets with diapers, diaper rash ointment, powder, wipes

- Assist and advise on child proofing ideas
- Go along with her to put together the baby registry
- Help pack hospital bag in the second trimester
- Help her buy essentials covered in her shopping list
- Wash, fold and put away newborn clothing
- Help her stock and pack cupboards and refrigerator for after delivery
- Help clean and clear areas like wardrobes and cupboards to make space for packing baby clothes, gear and equipment and additional groceries
- Purchase a white board, schedule or log books to help keep her organized

Assistance while MoM is hospitalized

- Put in car seats if you have experience with this
- Cook and freeze meals for the family to eat when MoM is on bed rest, in the hospital and after delivery e.g. meals that the family like, easy cook homemade foods, crock pot recipes, lasagna and casseroles
- Have house clean and orderly when she goes to the hospital e.g. laundry, put out the garbage, cupboards stocked
- Coordinate the services of the friends and family members that volunteered to assist with the babies and household chores after babies are born
- Organise help for the older children while MoM is at the hospital.
- Organize a 'welcome home MoM and babies' or 'congratulations' banner or a surprise for MoM

12

The babies are here!

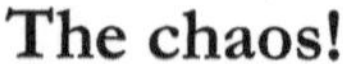

The chaos!

For the first week, mastering breastfeeding was really hard and hearing babies screaming while you are trying to feed another was no help. My son remained in the Neonatal Intensive Care Unit (NICU) for a week and the logistics of getting there alone was a feat as I was still very sore from my C-section and still a bit groggy from the anesthetic. Not to mention that seeing my son in the NICU attached to all those tubes was very depressing and terrifying.

The first month was really very hectic, overwhelming and mind boggling. Sleep deprivation was the order of the day. "How was I supposed to breastfeed 3 babies and still have time to do anything else like the bare necessities? You know like get out of bed, have breakfast and have a shower!"

I could barely find time to answer the phone or emails and I definitely did not want to see anyone who was not immediate family. Anyone in my house was an active "soldier" cooking, cleaning doing laundry, feeding or bathing babies, something, anything that could help get me some time or some sleep.

I had to give my friend with 5 year old triplets a call. I asked totally exasperated, "How in God's name did you survive this?"

Her response was just what I needed to carry on, "You will be just fine! I know you are more than capable. Just organize your troops and you will be just fine"!

-Author

The babies are here, and your calls and emails go unanswered but you would like to sneak a peek at her precious bundles. Think again! Unless you are an awfully close friend or a first degree relative do not try to visit within the first month. Many times, PoMs would like to have some time for their family to adjust to the new arrivals without having a constant flow of visitors. An email of congratulations or a phone call, with an offer to stop by as soon as they are up to visitors is much better during the first few weeks after birth. If your calls go unanswered call or email again a few weeks later. After the first 3 months you can visit at the PoMs convenience. Remember no one wants you to appear unknowingly in their chaotic home, with them looking unkempt and frazzled.

So the MoM has not asked you to help her and you are wondering if she needs help? The birth of her babies starts a period of mental anguish, anxiety and sleep deprivation and extra well placed offers of help is always welcomed. From my Survey of MoMs, some of the most common needs of PoMs when the babies arrive are:

- Meal preparation for adults
- Night assistance e.g. night feeding
- Assistance with chores e.g. laundry, folding clothes, washing and sterilizing bottles, cleaning
- Running errands e.g. running to the grocery
- Anything that would allow her to have a shower and catch a nap!

Here are some direct quotes from MoMs to prospective helpers of MoMs from my Survey of MoMs:

- "Anything helps, from laundry, to feedings, to all basic care of the little ones, cleaning around the home, help her with her own meals at times. I had all this help for the first year and it was amazing."

- "It was scary. When you can, go over and take care of them so she can sleep."
- "Take a night shift during the first weeks home. Help with meals or laundry. Help with the older one. Just be there to help!"
- "I'd say meals, cleaning and feedings so she can catch up on some zzzz's. At least that's what I wish I'd have had!"
- "Just be there and ask her what she needs."
- "Just ask...or help with errands, housework, etc....Maybe give her a break, out of the house!"
- "Support, cleaning and just let her know you are there to help!"
- "There will always be something to do! Once her babies come, I'm sure she will have lots for you to help and support her with."
- "Be there to help her keep her sanity!"
- "It is the little things that help tremendously e.g. wash bottles, fold the laundry, offer to feed and change babies."
- "Be there for her, even when she doesn't ask."
- "Make her easy to cook/reheat healthy meals. My mom brought a few weeks worth of meals along with healthy snacks and it was so nice not to have to worry about trying to cook."
- "She will need help with everything especially cooking and shopping and helping with the babies. You will be a godsend."
- "My friends made meals for us - which I froze. That was so helpful!"
- "I needed help washing bottles, cooking etc. Help with anything that didn't involve sleeping, showering or breast feeding. I was a mess for several weeks. The lack of sleep is horrible."
- "Set up a diaper brigade for a year. It was such a blessing to have diapers and wipes taken care of during that time. They would arrive on our doorstep each week."
- "Food and laundry! Having meals brought to me and ready to go was invaluable to me when my triplets were first home."

- "Food, cleaning, laundry, and watch the kids so she can shower and nap. If you can get people to donate diapers that's always great!"

Some periods in the life of a MoM are more stressful and hectic than others and warrant more assistance than other times. MoMs can always use an extra pair of hands at the right time. Many times, we just don't know how to ask for the help that we need. There will be many opportunities when new MoMs will need assistance and offers to assist will be greatly appreciated. These include:

- First few weeks
- Baby(ies) in the NICU
- Death of a child
- Diagnosis of special condition of a child
- First 3 months
- Breast feeding
- Night time
- Teething time
- Crawling and walking babies
- Babies begin moving around
- Financial Hardship
- Emotional periods
- Post Partum Depression
- Marital stress
- Low on supplies e.g. baby supplies, groceries
- Siblings are acting up

The possibility of acceptance of assistance may be greater around these times. These times should be triggers for you to offer your specific assistance or ask her what she needs to make this period less stressful.

13

Parting Words

Thank you for taking the time to read and understand what your friend/relative is going through while she is pregnant with multiples. I told you it was a lot of work! Just imagine pregnancy is the easy part! Reading this book has placed you in a far more advantageous position than her other friends and relatives. Now you know of the many instances throughout her pregnancy where she will need some assistance. Some expectant MoMs may have many offers to help, but I can tell you not all help is valuable.

Carrying multiples will be much less overwhelming if she has a team of genuine, reliable and trustworthy helpers at her side. Any effort to decrease her level of emotional and physical stress serves to enhance her physical condition and positively impact her growing babies. The insight and the tips I gave to you in this book will help you better understand and be proactive in giving the kind of help that she needs through her successful multiples pregnancy.

A word of caution; some people are less than enthusiastic to ask for or even accept help. She may not realize that she needs the assistance or may be trying to prove that she can be strong and do everything herself like I was. I beg you to be patient. Remember some people are very independent, organized and private and may not want too many family members or friends around. Even if she refuses to accept physical help or emotional support you can try to engage her in some fun and relaxation activities which will help her more than she knows it.

Once the babies arrive the family will need even more help. Some of the things mentioned in this book can be continued after their birth as well like providing emotional support, helping with chores and errands, baby shopping, giving a financial contribution, fun and relaxation, emotional support and of course helping with the babies. There is always the need for extra hands at feeding, photography, laundry, errand running, bath time and caring for other children/siblings to name just a few areas. The less she has to worry about with her babies the better for her. It will help her keep her sanity!

My last pieces of advice for you is just get out there and start helping your friend/relative and have fun doing it!

Appendix 1

Gathering Perspectives

To help give you a wider perspective in this book, I conducted a few informal surveys on present and expectant MoMs and on their friends and relatives and my friends and relatives. More specifically:

(i) To obtain the perspectives and experiences of MoMs I participated in online chats and actual conversations with present and expectant PoMs and administered an online survey to 100 MoMs of twins, triplets or quadruplets called Fun being pregnant with multiples- Is it or isn't it? These surveys provided some insight into issues like:

- Questions on her mind while pregnant
- Issues and concerns during her pregnancy
- What she did for fun during pregnancy
- Assistance that she needed from other persons while pregnant
- Her pregnancy experience
- Indications on the best and most useful gifts for her specific situation
- Silly questions that people ask expectant MoMs

(ii) To obtain the concerns and questions of the friends and relatives of expectant MoMs, I participated in online chats and actual conversations with the friends and relatives of PoMs and my friends and relatives. The informal survey was called 'The survey of present and prospective helpers to MoMs. The information gathered from this give a clearer understanding of:

- Questions asked by relatives and friends of PoMs
- Things that they would like to know about multiple pregnancy
- What type of assistance they have or are willing to provide to an expectant MoM?
- Issues on purchasing for an expectant MoM

Appendix 2

List of possible questions on the expectant MoMs mind

About herself

- Can I cope with this?

- How much weight do I need to gain?

- What do I need to eat to meet my nutritional needs for all of us?

- Will I be on bed rest?

- How will I breast feed them?

- How will I deal with the lack of sleep when they are born?

- How will I feel during this pregnancy?

- How well or ill will I feel for the next few months?

- What can I do to make everything go as smoothly as possible?

- How long will I be able to work during this pregnancy?

- Can I successfully carry more than one baby?

- I've had miscarriages before, how can I make this situation different?

- Should I terminate one baby's life to give the other(s) a greater chance at survival?

- How do you prepare for the arrival of more than one baby?

- Is feeling anxious/ nervous normal?

- Will asking for help make me seem incompetent or vulnerable?

- How long will I take to recover fully from my C-section?

- How will this impact on my lifestyle and the day to day routines of work, recreation and home?

- How will my life change?

- Will I lose my baby weight?

- What will my post pregnancy body look like?

- Does or will my husband still find me attractive?

- Where can I find people that I can relate to, like support groups and other expectant MoMs?

About her babies

- Will they be premature?
- Will they all survive?
- Will they have any disabilities/special needs?
- What size will my babies be?
- Will any of them need to stay in the Neonatal Intensive care Unit (NICU?)
- What's it like having your baby(ies) in the NICU?
- How does the logistics of having babies at home and in the NICU work e.g. breastfeeding?

Other

- Can we handle this financially?
- What is my best anesthetic option for delivery?
- Is my house large enough?
- Is my car large enough?
- What and how many items to buy?
- How do I share the news with friends and family?
- When and how do I share the news with my boss or work colleagues?
- How is this going to affect my relationship/ marriage?
- How much leave am I entitled too?
- Am I eligible for any financial entitlements?
- Where do I get coupons, discounts, and freebies for multiple births?
- How does my significant other really feel about these babies?
- Will friends and family members who promised to help really keep their word?

Appendix 3

Tips for Planning a Baby Shower for Twins, Triplets and More

Having multiples, whether it is to first time or experienced parents, is definitely a time for celebration. You can be the one to make it tons of fun for the expectant parents with a baby shower. Although a lot of fun, it is not without contention how the shower should be planned and whether it should be for new MoMs only, a co-ed event, before or after the birth of the babies, a traditional baby shower, what gift(s) to buy, who should be invited and the list goes on. Planning a shower for the mommy to be of multiples is similar to that for a single birth but with a twist and some additional important considerations. Let me give you some tips to help make this a fun and memorable experience for the expectant parents.

Anyone can host the baby shower

- Whether you are a friend, a relative or a co-worker, you can have a shower for the expectant MoM. These days, showers can be planned by friends, relatives, her mother, mother-in-law, co-workers, the expectant mother's best girl friends, neighbors or a group to which she belongs - you name it! Basically, anyone who wants to help her share her good news and get some well needed advice, gifts and best wishes can host the baby shower. The expectant MoM will be also happy with more than one event if it is thoughtfully planned and coordinated and if she is physically capable to attend.

Consult with MoM

- The key to a successful baby shower is to consult with the expectant MoM to ensure her needs and wishes are considered e.g. who she may want to invite, the type of shower she wants, when she wants it etc. There are some matters that may be thought to be tradition and should not be changed, however these matters are as important as she makes them.

- Also be sure to ask about the items that she has already purchased if she does not have a baby registry, that way guests can get her items that she does not have yet.

- Be sure to ask if there are other persons that are hosting any other baby showers for her to avoid scheduling conflicts and facilitate synchronization if necessary. Remember her time is limited so a meaningful and thoughtful event is deserved.

Give her the type of shower she wants or needs

- Be sure to ask MoM if she has any preferences for the type of shower before you start planning. Because multiples arrive earlier the expectant MoM may have started her shopping earlier or friends and family may have pitched in earlier. This can determine the type of shower she would like to have. Some ideas include:

- Traditional shower - This is the most common type of shower and is best timed when she does not have all her supplies, equipment and clothes yet. Her friends and family can help with her purchases by bringing thoughtful and useful gifts

- Diaper drive - Multiples use a lot of diapers! If she already has all her toys, equipment and supplies she may prefer a diaper drive where guests provide a variety of diapers in various sizes and wipes. Note: Confirm with her which is her diaper preference - disposable or cloth before you purchase

- Food drive - After the babies arrive, MoM may not have the time to cook meals for her family. If she foresees that meals will be her biggest challenge, she may prefer a food drive where her friends can cook, buy or put together ready to reheat meals to relieve her of meal planning for the first few weeks. Make sure she has the freezer space for this or organize a delivery schedule as they are needed.

- Pampering shower - If she already has all the gear and equipment for her babies or needs to be the center of attention until the babies arrive, this is a good idea. This is all about the expectant MoM and not about the babies. Spa services can be provided at the location of the shower e.g. prenatal massage, manicures, pedicures. Or gifts can be about pampering MoM while pregnant or after she has her babies e.g. comfortable pajamas, body care items, gift certificates for spa services etc.

Check with her for invitees

- This is not your decision and your views on the matter don't really count. The expectant MoM should decide who she would like to attend. Some may like to have the dad to be and her other children in attendance, her mother and/or mother-in-law or a co-ed shower. Ensure that you check with her to make certain that everyone she deems important enough to share her day with her are invited and to avoid inviting persons that she may not care to include.

Timing is everything

- Before the third trimester - In the case of multiples the shower should be held sooner than for a mom of a singleton. The consideration of discomfort, bed rest and preterm labor is a reality in this case that can render your planning effort futile. The late second trimester is the ideal time.
- Never throw a surprise baby shower - Expectant MoMs may have a more difficult pregnancy, more doctors' visits and more rest in their schedule. You must consult with her to find out what her schedule is like and how she is feeling so she can look her best for the occasion!
- The shower should be at a reasonable time of the day as determined by the expectant MoM and for only a few hours.
- An arrival shower is an option - A meet and greet the babies after

the birth is also a consideration. Ask her views on this. Some MoMs may prefer this especially if they are having a difficult pregnancy or are on bed rest. The advantage here is that guests can bring gifts specific to her needs after birth. The babies will now become the center of attraction of the event.

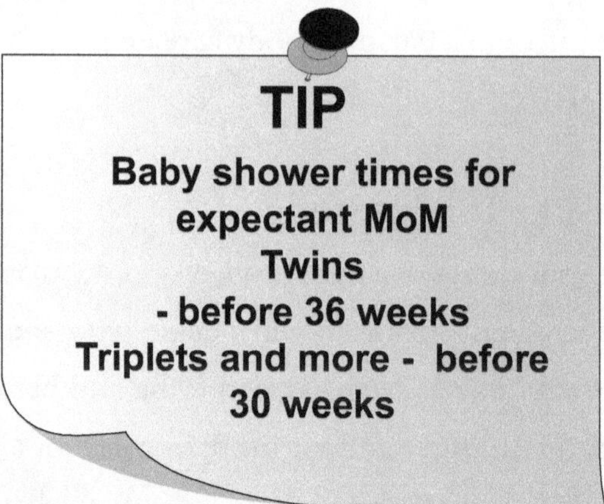

Choose a comfortable location

- The location should be convenient to the expectant MoM as her mobility may be limited. So, forget the restaurant and the club, her home is a better option or the home of a friend or relative near by.
- Comfortable seating, like a recliner for the expectant MoM, is a necessity as she may not be able to sit comfortably for long periods of time. Preferably organize semi reclined seating or a leg rest.
- Ensure that the location chosen can hold the number of guests and the gifts as well. Also, it should be convenient for her to get back to her home or bed with her gifts packed away.

There should be nothing for MoM to do

- The guests and organizers should do everything from planning to the cleaning up, the entertaining and even packing away gifts. The expectant MoM's only task should be to show up.

Don't break the bank

- Food and drinks can be approximately 40-50% of the budgeted expenses so cost cutting here I know will be appreciated. A potluck where friends and family bring the food, finger foods, cake and drinks will be a huge saving.
- Using her home, offering your home or using that of a close friend will avoid the cost of a restaurant or rental of an event location.
- Bulk buying decorations can keep costs down.
- Utilizing online services to send invitations for the younger and the tech savvy while using the traditional mail service for the older and less tech savvy participants like her grandmother!
- You are not obligated to purchase double and triple your budget because she is expecting multiples. You can be creative in your gift buying.

Give thoughtful and useful gifts

- Encourage her to create a baby registry. It makes life easier for both the expectant MoM and her friends and relatives to choose gifts. It ensures that she gets what she wants, avoids duplication and is easy for out of town guests. If there is no registry here are some options:
    - Check with her to see what she would like or what she already has
    - Choose a larger ticket item and have guests contribute to it e.g. strollers, cribs, furniture
    - Create themed gift baskets and let guests contribute either money or items towards it e.g. baby bedtime basket, bath time bundle, diapering and changing supplies etc.
    - Buy multiples of items so you don't have to consider each child individually e.g. multiple packs of socks, onesies etc.
    - Buy multiples specific gifts

- Make diaper cakes - nicely wrapped diapers adorned with some other baby necessities

Make a multiples theme work for you

- Invitations
- Be sure to include that she is expecting multiples and the gender of the babies if she is sharing that type of information.
- Be sure to include all the information in them: who, what, where, when, RSVP instructions and if she is registered anywhere for baby gifts.
- Send the invitations 3-6 weeks in advance depending on the group of invitees. You must give them enough time to work it into their schedule and to shop for the perfect gift.

Theme, décor, favors

- The shower can have a multiples specific theme e.g. twin or triplet related. e.g. three peas in a pod, Noah's Ark 2 by 2 concept, Goldilocks and the three bears, two of a kind etc.

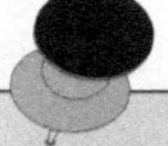

TIP

Multiples Baby shower ideas For ideas on multiples themes, with matching baby shower decorations, invitations, thank you cards, banners and tableware and favors- check www.babyshowerstuff.com

- The décor, invitations, favors etc. can all be worked into your theme.
- Be creative if it does not have to break the bank - balloons grouped by color to represent gender, toys and décor or streamers in groups of two or three to represent twins or triplets etc.

Games

- Games are usually a highlight of the event for many. Know your audience and keep it simple e.g. let guests cut a piece of ribbon to the estimated size of her belly, or teams can dress three dolls (triplets) with one hand and the team with the shortest time wins.
- Use prizes as incentives like snacks, body care products etc.
- There are tons of games on the internet for baby showers for twins and triplets.

Appendix 4

Tips for Buying for Twins, Triplets and More

Purchasing items for a mother of one baby can be daunting as can be buying for more than one baby. The parents of multiples have multiple times the fun, stress and costs of a mother with a single baby. You can help offset some of their expenses by giving some thoughtful and creative gifts. Many MoMs find themselves stumped in stores as they venture to purchase items and gifts for their little ones. Some of them receive numerous phone calls from friends and family members around Christmas and birthday time when people are shopping for gifts for these little ones.

Ask PoMs what they and the babies need

- Asking what they want ensures that your money is well spent on something that will be of definite use to the children or their parents.

Buy practical things

- Consider practical things when looking for a gift from babies up to two years old

Diapers, wipes, formula, onesies, sleepers, bath time products

- This avoids a stockpile of items that may hardly be used

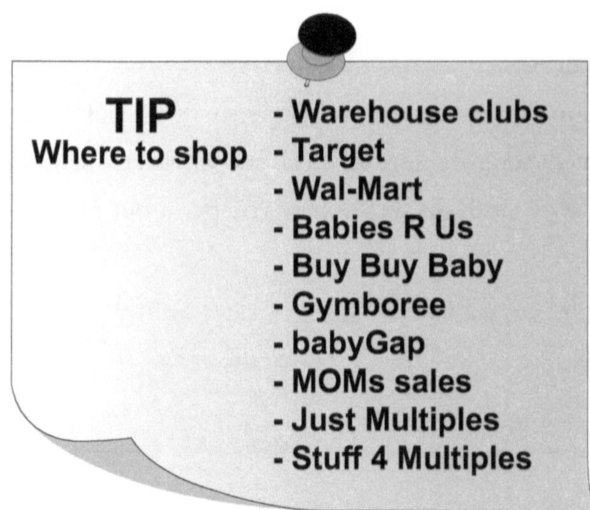

Buy practical things

- Consider practical things when looking for a gift from babies up to two years old - Diapers, wipes, formula, onesies, sleepers, bath time products
- This avoids a stockpile of items that may hardly be used

Convenience

There are tons of items put on this earth to make the life of a MoM easier. We want anything that will give us an extra few minutes, less noise, less wailing, more sleep time for the babies, more rest time for us and happy babies!! Here are some great gift ideas I've sourced from my own experience and fellow MoMs.

- Easier feeding and to free our hands - boppy pillows, nursing pillows, bottle props, podee bottles, feeding time helpers
- To free our hands and soothe babies - swings, bouncy chairs
- Less trips to the baby store and supermarket - gift basket with bath essentials, laundry essentials, feeding essentials
- To do laundry less frequently - a lot of crib sheets, sleepers/footed pajamas, onesies, receiving blankets
- Less trips to the nursery - baby monitor, diapering essentials basket

Diaper drive

- A collection of various sizes of diapers will be useful; wipes can also be included here. Be sure to find out whether MoM will be using disposable or cloth diapers before you go about purchasing diapers for her
- Buy in bulk
- Go online
- Use coupons

> **Diapers, diapers and more diapers!**
> **On average a baby uses 8-10 disposable diapers a day during the first year.**
> **Monthly usage**
> **Singleton - 240-300 diapers**
> **Twins   - 480-600 diapers**
> **Triplets   - 720-900 diapers**

Determine number of items

- Don't buy two or three toys/ equipment unless requested.

- There are some items deemed as necessities and MoM will need the number to match her babies while there are items that can be shared or rotated. Many MoMs end up rotating items. So, varieties of things may be better e.g. a swing, a bouncy chair etc.

- Buy one and see how the babies respond to it before purchasing multiples of them e.g. swings, bouncy chairs, exersaucer, walkers etc.

- Gifts that are multiples of items are well suited for this predicament e.g. multiple packs of onesies, bibs, socks, neutral colored sleepers.

Don't break the bank/ budget

- You must consider each baby but you are not obligated to double or triple your budget. If you are on a tight budget you can purchase one item or a group of items that they all can use.

Most frequently asked question when purchasing for multiples - "How much items to buy?"

Buying clothes

- Although the children were born together, they are usually different sizes. The remedy is to purchase a few items of different sizes. Also purchase clothes two to three sizes larger so MoM can have it for longer use and they can pass it along as well

- MoMs may or may not use clothes to differentiate between her children. So, ask her on her preference of coordinated or matching outfits: same color different style, same style but different color, different altogether, a color for a particular child, type of clothing per child etc. This not a consideration when purchasing for a singleton, so ask.

Preemie sized clothing

- Consult with her before purchasing

- The size of multiple birth babies poses a challenge in the early days

- Multiples are usually smaller than the average singleton, may have special requirements or there may be hospital guidelines that may limit their clothing options

- Although they may be premature at birth, they may only use preemie sized clothing for a very short time

- Many stores are starting to offer preemie sized clothing which makes

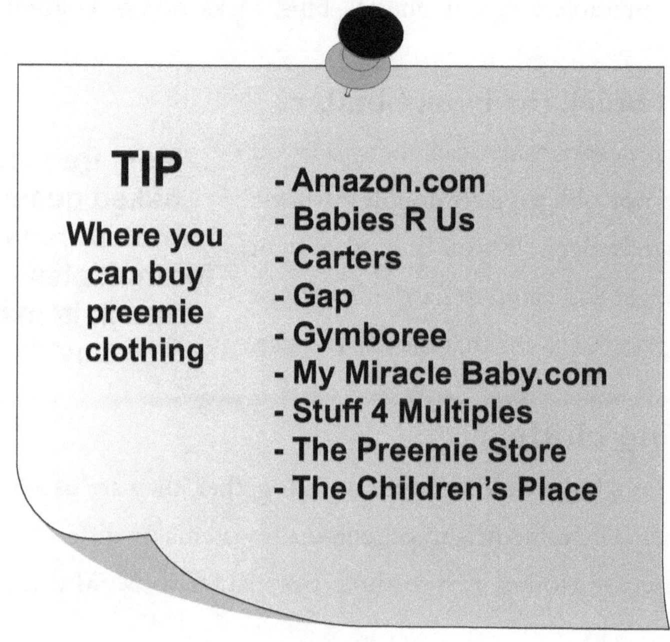

it much easier to find things for smaller than average babies

- Some major stores have also started selling preemie lines; however, they aren't always available in the stores. Online purchasing may be a good option.

Large items

- Consult with the expectant MoM on larger items etc. to ensure they carry the specifications that she needs before purchasing the items, as she may have additional concerns and considerations. For example:
    - o Cribs - larger to hold more than one baby or not
    - o Strollers - side by side vs. tandem
    - o Car seats - can they fit in their present vehicles
    - o Furniture e.g. changing tables, rockers - may need dual purpose to save space

Needs in stages

- To prevent clutter in our homes there are items that are bought in stages. So instead of stockpiling these items, you have the opportunity to fulfill MoMs needs for the following at various times:
    - o Diapers - children outgrow them quickly
    - o Clothes - children may be the same age but not the same size
    - o Food items - dietary needs and preferences change or allergies develop
    - o Toys - developmentally appropriate

Storage considerations

- It may be wiser to purchase certain larger items when needed, as storage of multiples of large items may be an issue e.g. high chairs, wagons, gates, playpens

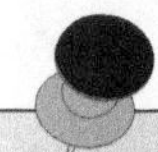

Specialized items

- If you would like to purchase specialized items - Google search specialized twin and triplet items
- Personalized clothes, bibs, tops, t-shirts for babies and adults, hats are options

Buying toys

- Birth to two years - different variations of the same category of gift and approximately the same size. e.g. stuffed animal - bear, dog, frog
- Buy multiples of small toys e.g. dolls, bears, balls

Save receipts

- Save boxes and receipts to facilitate returns. Sometimes MoM may receive duplicates of items, that may be impractical to her specific needs, items that the children may have an allergic reaction to and may need to return them

Discounts

- Be sure to ask for discounts when purchasing multiples of the same item

Gift baskets

- You can put together any amount or type of items that you would like in a gift basket for the babies or for MoM. It can collectively have something in common e.g. bedtime, bathtime, safety, books, fruits, food, necessities, spa

- Bath - baby shampoo, liquid soap, in a bathtub

Bulk buying

- The saying "cheaper by the dozen" applies here. Formula, bottles, pacifiers, diapers, wipes and baby food are used in great quantities so purchasing in bulk will be a tremendous cost saving. The downside here is that babies preferences and needs change frequently and you will not want to invest in a lot of an item if this happens

Gently used

- Ask the expectant MoM about her views on gently used items. You can pick up a few items like toys and equipment. These are pretty expensive these days and children outgrow them quickly. Garage sales, consignment and thrift stores can provide many much needed items and not break the bank.

Appendix 5

Registry Checklist for Multiples

I found this list of items quite helpful while checking around and shopping for my babies' gear and wear. This will give an idea of what needs to be purchased and how many.

Furniture/ bedding

Cribs (babies may be able to share in the beginning, but they start wriggling around pretty quickly, so 1 per baby)

Crib mattresses (1 per baby) and covers

2–3 fitted crib sheets (per crib)

Dresser

Changing table

Gear

High chairs (1 per baby)

Swing (buy 1 and see if you need more down the line)

Bouncer seat or rocker (you may be able to get away with having just 1 here, too)

Car seats (1 per baby/no skimping here!)

Car window shade

Stroller (choose one that can accommodate all of your babies)

Umbrella stroller (You only really need one stroller, but it's good to also have an umbrella stroller for travel.)

Baby slings or carriers

Diaper bag

Changing mat (just get 1 of these)

Diaper pail and liner

Activity mat (get a big one that can accommodate all of your babies)

Safety/health

Baby monitor

Pacifiers

Thermometer

Nasal aspirator

Baby nail clippers

First-aid kit

Infant bathtub

2 hooded bath towels per baby

4 washcloths per baby

Baby shampoo and wash

Brush and comb set

Diaper rash cream

Diapers (start with at least 2 cases of newborn size)

Clothing

4–6 undershirts per baby

4–6 receiving blankets per baby

4–6 long-sleeved onesies per baby

4 sleep sacks per baby

Caps/mittens

Feeding

Breast pump

Multiples nursing pillow

4–8 bibs per baby

Burp cloths

10–16 bottles per baby

Insulated bottle tote

Bottle brush

Bottle sterilizer

Bottle warmers

Dishwasher caddy

Excerpted from The Bump : Registry for Multiples

Suggested Readings and Bibliography

Adams, Victoria. Triplets? Relax - Tips to Guide you through the first year Sanity intact. Victoria Adams, 2014

Blickley, Leigh. Celebrity Twins: 23 Stars You Didn't Know Were Twins. Last modified March 2013. http://www.huffingtonpost.com/2012/11/28/celebrity-twins-23-stars-you-may-not-have-known-were-a-twin-photos_n_2198990.html#slide=1816142

Fierro, Pamela. Mommy Rescue Guide - Twins Triplets and More - Life Saving Techniques and Advice for Surviving Life with Multiples. Adams Media, 2008

Fierro, Pamela. Twin Baby Shower - Who to Invite to a Baby Shower for Twins or Multiples. Last modified April 17, 2014. http://multiples.about.com/od/pregnancy/a/twinbabyshower.htm

Fierro, Pamela. Top 11 Celebrity Dads of Twins: Actors. Last Modified March 25, 2014. http://multiples.about.com/od/celebrities/tp/famousactordadoftwins.htm

Fierro, Pamela. Top 23 Celebrity Mothers of Twins. Last modified May 11, 2014 http://multiples.about.com/od/celebrities/tp/famoustwinmom.htm

Fierro, Pamela. Celebrity Twins: Who Knew? These Celebs Are Also Twins. Last modified April 09, 2014. http://multiples.about.com/od/celebrities/tp/celebritysecrettwins.htm

Lorenz, Lynn. The Multiples Manual - Preparing and Caring for Twins or Triplets - Pregnancy to Preschool. Just Multiples.com, 2007

Luke, Barbara and T Eberlien. When You're Expecting Twins, Triplets or Quads. William Morrow Paperbacks, 2010

Lyons, Elizabeth. Ready or Not...Here We Come! The Real Experts' Guide to the First Year with Twins. Finn-Phyllis Press, 2007

Martin JA, BE Hamilton, MJK Osterman et al. National Vital Statistics Reports, Volume 68, Number 13- Births: Final Data for 2018. Division of Vital Statistics. November 27 2019. https://www.cdc.gov/nchs/data/nvsr/nvsr68/nvsr68_13-508.pdf

Rawlinson, Joe. Dad's Guide to Twins: How to Survive the Twin Pregnancy and Prepare for your Twins. Texadoro LLC, 2013

Scalise, Dagmara. Twin Sense - A Sanity Saving Guide to Raising Twins from Pregnancy through the First Year. AMACOM, 2008

Tinglof, Christina Baglivi. Double Duty: The Parents' Guide to Raising Twins, from Pregnancy Through the School Years (2nd edition). McGraw-Hill, 2009

"A Child Born in 2012 Will Cost $241,080 to Raise According to USDA Report," USDA News Release. August 13, 2013. http://www.usda.gov/wps/portal/usda/usdahome?contentid=2013/08/0160.xml

"Child Trends Databank." (2015). Preterm births. Available at: https://www.childtrends.org/wp-content/uploads/2015/06/indicator_1434209915.291.html

"Depression in Pregnancy." American Pregnancy Association. Last modified January 2013. http://americanpregnancy.org/pregnancy-health/depressionduringpregnancy.html

"Divorce and the Multiple Birth Family". MOST (Mothers of Supertwins) http://www.mostonline.org/facts_divorcesurvey.htm

"Incidence of Twins by Twin Type" Twins Magazine https://twins-magazine.com/incidence-of-twins-by-twin-type/

"Supertwins101." MOST (Mothers of Supertwins) http://www.mostonline.org/faq_expecting.htm

"Weight Gain During Pregnancy" March of Dimes - https://www.marchofdimes.org/pregnancy/weight-gain-during-pregnancy.aspx

Other Useful Information

Multiples Support Groups and websites

ABC-Club (Germany)

Association Jumeaux (Switzerland)

Australian Multiple Birth Association (AMBA)

Finnish Multiple Births Association (Finland):

International Council of Multiple Birth Organisation (ICOMBO)

Irish Multiple Births Associations (Ireland)

International Society for Twin Studies

International Twins Association, Inc.

Japanese Association of Twins' Mothers (Japan)

Jumeaux et plus, l'Association Fédération (France)

Multifamilias (Argentina)

Multiple Births Canada/Naissances Multiples Canada (MBC)

Multiple Births Foundation (UK)

Multiple Births Foundation (Srilanka)

Multiples New Zealand

Norwegian Organization (Norway)

Twinstrust (England):

Bereavement Support

Center for Loss in Multiple Birth (CLIMB, Inc.)

The Lone Twin Network

SIDS Alliance, Inc.

Twinless Twins Support Group, International (US)

General websites with information for MoMs

Babycenter - https://www.babycenter.com/

Parenting - https://www.parenting.com/

RaisingMultiples - https://www.raisingmultiples.org/

Twin Pregnancy and Beyond - https://www.twin-pregnancy-and-beyond.com

The bump - https://www.thebump.com/

What to expect - https://www.whattoexpect.com/

Twin Stuff - https://twinstuff.com/

Parenting and Multiples Magazines for her

TWINS

American Baby

Parenting

Multiples

Babytalk

List of discounts and freebies

www.babycenter.com/freestuff/

www.babychatter.com

www.preemietwins.com/twinsfreestuff.htm

www.twinslist.org/freebie.htm

www.mostonline.org/membersonly/company.htm

www.verywellfamily.com/top-discounts-freebies-for-twinsmultiples

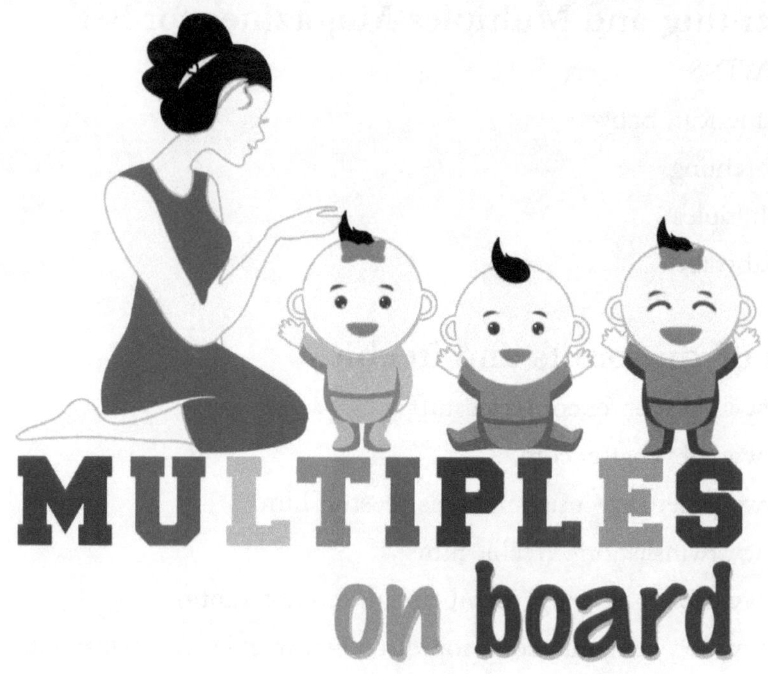
MULTIPLES
on board

About the Author

Sharlene Gittens-Francis BSc., MBA is the mother of triplets (two girls and one boy) and has worked in various fields of sales, project management, business development and market research in Trinidad and Tobago. These days this Caribbean woman is a wife, mother, friend, chef, chauffeur, interior decorator, janitor, mediator, party planner, a business and research consultant, and is managing one of the biggest projects of her life – Raising her Triplets.

This busy mother of multiples accepted the help of friends and family members even though she did not want to admit she needed it during her pregnancy. In fact, she attributes this to her successful and stress free multiple pregnancy.

The love, support and help that she received from her friends and family during her pregnancy has been the inspiration for her social networking site Multiples on Board and her book – **She's Expecting Multiples**. She has devoted time to sharing her experience as a MoM and expertise as a researcher to help the friends and family members get on board.

90-DAY
Mediterranean Diet
1500-CALORIE

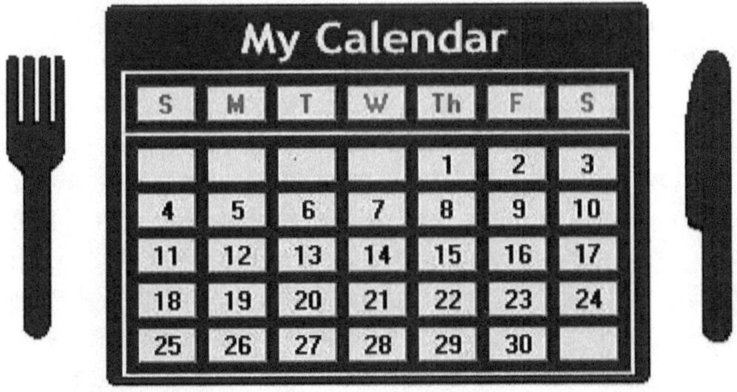

Vincent Antonetti, PhD
Tina Hudson, M.S.

NoPaperPress™

NOTE: At publication, the off-the-shelf foods used in portions of this book were widely available in most supermarkets. But food products come and go. So if there is a frozen entrée or soup selection in this diet that is out of stock, or that's been discontinued, or perhaps that you don't like, or that you forgot to pick up while shopping, please substitute another food that has **approximately** the same caloric value and nutritional content. In this regard, many dieters have found the foods listed in the Appendices at the end of this book to be very helpful.

PREFACE

In 1958, Dr. Ancel Keys, a highly-regarded scientist at the University of Minnesota, started a landmark research project of healthy middle-aged men called The Seven Countries Study[1]. The project lasted decades and included men living in Greece, Italy, Yugoslavia, the Netherlands, Finland, and the United States. His findings supported previous studies that pointed to saturated fats as the cause of the arterial blockages that resulted in heart disease and heart attacks. But he also found that in Mediterranean countries, such as Greece and Italy, heart disease was not as prevalent and caused fewer deaths than in northern Europe and the United States. Dr. Keys was the first to advocate the health implications of a Mediterranean-style diet.

Generally speaking the Mediterranean diet is a way of eating based on the long-established cuisine of the countries bordering the Mediterranean Sea. The diet typically contains lots of vegetables, fruits, whole grain breads, beans, seafood, nut and seeds, olive oil and red wine. Plant-based foods are central to the diet. But moderate amounts of dairy, seafood, poultry and eggs are also important in the Mediterranean Diet. In contrast, red meat is eaten infrequently.

Healthy fats are a mainstay of a Mediterranean diet and are consumed instead of unhealthy saturated and trans fats which contribute to heart disease. Olive oil is the primary source of added fat in a Mediterranean diet. Olive oil is a monounsaturated fat, which has been found to lower total cholesterol and LDL (or "bad") cholesterol levels. Nuts and seeds also contain monounsaturated fat.

Seafood is also important in the Mediterranean diet. Fatty fish such as mackerel, herring, sardines, albacore tuna, salmon and lake trout, all rich in omega-3 fatty acids, a type of polyunsaturated fat that is thought to reduce inflammation in humans. Omega-3 fatty acids also help to decrease triglycerides, reduce blood clotting, and decrease the risk of stroke and congestive heart failure. A typical Mediterranean diet allows red wine - but only in moderation.

Research has shown that the Mediterranean Diet is by far one of the healthiest in the world. It's important to note that the Mediterranean Diet in this book is also a **Reducing Diet** and therefore shows the caloric value of the foods in the diet. In fact, what makes the Mediterranean Diet in this book different is the emphasis on calorie control which is what leads directly to weight loss.

The version of the Mediterranean Diet in this book has been modified slightly to be consistent with American dietary patterns, food preferences and calorie control.

Note that Vince (the primary author) is three-quarters Italian and Tina's mother was of Italian decent. This is the diet we both grew up eating.

Vince Antonetti & Tina Hudson
July 2020

1. Keys, Ancel. "Coronary problems in seven countries." Circulation 41.1 (1970): 186-195.

CONTENTS

1500 CALORIE MEAL PLANS

RECIPIES & DIET TIPS

Day 52 Recipe: Chicken Piccata
Day 53 Recipe: Pasta Primavera (160)
Day 54 Recipe: Grilled Scallops & Polenta
Day 55 Recipe: Hearty Vegetable Soup (162)
Day 56 Recipe: Frozen Chicken Dinner
Day 57 Recipe: Salmon with Mango Salsa (164)
Day 58 Recipe: Grilled Pork Chop with Orange
Day 59 Recipe: Fish Dinner Out (166)
Day 60 Recipe: Chicken Stew over Rice
Day 61 Recipe: Shrimp over Spaghetti (168)
Day 62 Recipe: Beef Burgundy
Day 63 Recipe: Chicken Cutlet (170)
Day 64 Recipe: Turkey Meatloaf
Day 65 Recipe: Frozen Fish Dinner (172)
Day 66 Recipe: Pita Pizza
Day 67 Recipe: Chicken Dinner Out (174)
Day 68 Recipe: Pork Medallions in Lime Sauce
Day 69 Recipe: Healthy Chicken Salad (176)
Day 70 Recipe: Baked Cod
Day 71 Recipe: Chicken Scaloppini (178)
Day 72 Recipe: Fish Dinner Out
Day 73 Recipe: Pasta Pomodoro (180)
Day 74 Recipe: Frozen Chicken Dinner
Day 75 Recipe: Mediterranean Chicken (182)
Day 76 Recipe: Grilled Scallops
Day 77 Recipe: Chicken with Peppers & Rice (184)
Day 78 Recipe: Trout with Lemon & Capers
Day 79 Recipe: Italian Food - Out (186)
Day 80 Recipe: Vegetable Chilli
Day 81 Recipe: Frozen Meat Dinner (188)
Day 82 Recipe: Chicken Salad
Day 83 Recipe: Hearty Lentil Stew (190)
Day 84 Recipe: Turkey Burger
Day 85 Recipe: Lo-Cal Meat Loaf (192)
Day 86 Recipe: Tuna & Bean Salad
Day 87 Recipe: Pasta and Veggies (194)
Day 88 Recipe: Frozen Chicken Dinner
Day 89 Recipe: Fish Stew (196)
Day 90 Recipe: Veal with Mushrooms & Tomato

The Best Weight-Loss Diets

According to the late Dr. Jean Mayer of Harvard University's Department of Nutrition, a really good weight-loss diet must have the following three characteristics:

1) The diet must provide you with an understanding of weight control as well as the knowledge you need to reduce your weight to the desired level.

2) The diet must help you remain healthy while you are losing weight.

3) The diet must lead you to a healthier way of eating and exercising that will, in the long term, help you keep off the weight you have lost.

The Mediterranean weight-loss diet featured in this book is a diet that is not only low calorie and reasonably low in fat, but is also nutritionally balanced. The *90-Day Mediterranean Diet*, however, does not meet all the criteria set forth above. While you will acquire some "dieting insight" and some idea of how much you can eat and still lose weight, you will not get a real understanding of weight control from this book. That's not its purpose. What you will get is a healthy diet – and a diet that if followed will promote weight loss. Think of the *90-Day Mediterranean Diet* as a quick fix, a healthy start that will get you on the right track – but it's not the long-term answer.

Long-term success is about developing both an understanding and a plan that will result in healthier eating and physical activity habits. For a through understanding and the guidance you need to succeed in the long term we recommend you read, *Weight Control - U.S. Edition* by Vincent Antonetti, Ph.D., another NoPaperPress book.

Begin with a Medical Exam

Everyone should at the very least have a medical assessment, or exam, before starting a weight loss diet. Why? You need to make sure your health will allow you to lower your caloric intake and increase your physical activity. The medical checkup may be as simple as a visit to a physician who is familiar with your medical history, or it may be a thorough physical exam. The physician conducting the medical exam should be made aware of and should approve the specific weight loss diet you're planning.

What's in This Book?

This book contains 90 Daily Menus and 90 delicious Recipes.

How Much Weight Will You Lose?

Weight loss occurs when your food energy intake is less than the total energy you expend. This difference in calories is referred to as your <u>calorie deficit</u>. How much weight you lose depends on the magnitude of your calorie deficit. Simple metabolic calculations make a rough estimate possible.

On the 90-Day Mediterranean Diet, <u>most women lose 18 to 28 lbs.</u>

On the 90-Day Mediterranean Diet , <u>most men lose 28 to 38 lbs.</u>

Smaller adults, older adults and less active adults might lose a bit less and larger adults, younger adults and more active adults often much more. Exactly how much weight you will lose depends on how much you weigh, your age and your activity level. Again, for the full story see *Weight Control - U.S. Edition* by Vincent Antonetti, Ph.D.

Guidelines for Healthy Eating

Even though most adults can get all the vitamins and minerals they need by merely consuming a variety of nutritious foods (from the fruit group, the vegetable group, the grains group, the meat and beans group, the milk group, and the oils group), many physicians recommend a daily multi-vitamin/mineral supplement – just in case you don't eat the way you should.

<u>Large Salad:</u> One of the dinner mainstays is a "Large Salad." Prepare your "Large Salad" in a bowl with a volume of at least 16 ounces, or 2 cups. First add about 1 cup of either green leaf lettuce, Romaine lettuce or a mesclun mix. Then add, as desired, another cup of other veggies such as broccoli, celery, cucumber, tomato, onion, peppers, spinach, or watercress. This vegetable combination will, on average, total about 40 Calories. You will be eating a "Large Salad" just about every day at dinnertime. Remember that variety is the key to a nutritious diet. So be sure to vary the ingredients of the salad. Top your large salad with <u>two tablespoons</u> of the salad dressing discussed below.

For a **"Small Salad"** use half the ingredients of the preceding large salad and half of the salad dressing on the next page.

Salad Dressing: Mix two tablespoons of extra virgin olive oil (Evoo) with one tablespoon of balsamic vinegar and one tablespoon of water. Add salt, pepper and any Italian herbs to taste. Whisk ingredients together. Shake well. Use half of the dressing on your large salad. Save the remainder in your fridge.

Your "Large Salad" with salad dressing will cost you roughly 150 Calories but will be packed with lots of health-giving vitamins, minerals and fiber. The "Small Salad" contains about 75 Calories.

Homemade Cooking Spray: Simply combine one part olive oil with one part water into a spray bottle. Shake well and spray! Cheap, low calorie and effective.

Soup: See Appendix C page 205 for a list of the soup permitted on this diet. To improve the taste of a canned soup, add a teaspoon of grated cheese before heating in a microwave oven. After heating, add ½ teaspoon of olive oil. Stir and serve. These additions total about 30 Calories but really enhance the taste.

About Bread: First understand that bread, more specifically whole-grain breads, are good sources of complex carbohydrates and dietary fiber, as well as several B vitamins (thiamin, riboflavin, niacin, and foliate), vitamin E, and minerals (iron, magnesium and selenium). In recent years, however, sliced bread loaves have gotten larger, as have the bread slices inside these loaves. Just a few years ago the standard slice of bread contained about 65 to 70 Calories – now most are 100 plus Calories.

The *90-Day Mediterranean Diet* requires whole-grain bread at 65 to 70 Calories per slice for breakfast toast. Quite a few bakers sell thin sliced or "light" sliced bread. The difficult part is finding a whole grain thin sliced or "light" bread (with about 70 Calories per slice). Whatever the brand, make sure the first word in the Ingredients list is "whole." "Pepperidge Farm Small Slice 100% Whole Wheat" is a good breakfast choice. It's whole grain, has 70 Calories per slice and it tastes good too.

For dinner find a good loaf of **Italian or French bread** and use about one ounce (80 Calories). <u>Hint</u>: Get the weight of the loaf from a label, or weigh it on a scale in the produce section of the store. Then estimate how many one ounce servings the loaf contains and slice accordingly.

Exchanging Foods

If there is a food listed in the *90-Day Mediterranean Diet* that you don't like, or perhaps that you forgot to pick up while shopping, you probably can exchange or substitute another food in its place – a technique used by dieticians. Exchanging a food listed in a diet for another food with approximately equal caloric value and nutritional content is the foundation of a successful long-term diet. Substitution possibilities are almost endless but have to be done carefully.

The easiest substitutions are those within the same food group, such as exchanging one vegetable variety for another, or a glass of milk for a cup of yogurt. More sophisticated exchanges cross food groups, for instance replacing 3½ ounces of turkey with a tablespoon of peanut butter spread on a piece of whole wheat bread. Both foods are complete protein and both contain about 175 Calories.

Refer to a good online calorie table. With some understanding and experience, you can use this table to help you substitute foods called for in the *Mediterranean Diet* with equal calorie foods from the same food group.

Breakfast: You may substitute any cereal for any other wholesome cereal. For example, if you're not crazy about having Shredded Wheat for breakfast, substitute Wheat Chex or Cheerios, etc. If you don't like the soft-boiled egg called for on Day 9, make yourself a scrambled egg instead. And if Cantaloupe is on the menu but is not in season, replace the cantaloupe with a half cup of orange juice.

Snacks: Again, where yogurt is specified you may substitute a 6-ounce glass of skim milk, but to maintain a nutritionally balanced diet keep this snack a dairy selection. Similarly, when fruit is on the agenda, you may select another type of fruit but do not stray from the fruit group. Nuts and popcorn can be interchanged at will. (Incidentally, you should buy a hot-air popper. They make great popcorn – which is high in fiber and makes a tasty and nutritious snack.)

Two Nights Off

Everyone deserves a break from the grind of preparing dinner after coming home from work. So the *90-Day Mediterranean Diet* gives you two days off per week! Notice that one night a week the diet calls for a frozen dinner and on a second night during the week you're encouraged to eat out. There are, however, some rules and caveats involved and these are covered in the next two sections.

Frozen Dinners

In general, a frozen dinner should not be a meal in itself. Make sure you add a salad, fruit, bread etc. The frozen dinner you choose should come with at least one cup of cooked vegetables. If your frozen dinner doesn't measure up, add your own frozen, fresh or canned vegetables. And look for dinners with no more than 800 mg of sodium. In addition, make sure the dinner you choose has no more than 30 percent of the daily value for total fat. Appendix A page 198 lists almost 150 frozen dinner entrees.

And on the days when a frozen dinner is specified, you will also be given a calorie goal for the frozen dinner. For example, Day 5 calls for frozen fish dinner with a maximum allowable 300 Calories. If you choose a frozen fish dinner that contains less than 300 Calories, you may spend the unused calories any way you wish.

Moreover, on those nights when you just don't have the energy or time to cook, you can always substitute a frozen dinner for the entree listed in the meal plan. For example, Day 1 calls for Chicken with Peppers and Onions for dinner. The total calorie count for dinner is 500. In place of the Day 1 calls for Chicken with Peppers and Onions, any combination of a frozen chicken dinner and side dishes (salads, etc) with a total calorie content close to 500 would be an acceptable, albeit not as tasty, an alternative.

Eating Out

You may eat out once a week. When you're on a diet, however, eating in a restaurant can be a challenge, because most restaurant portions are huge, and can easily total more than 1,000 Calories. On the *90-Day Mediterranean Diet*, a dinner type (i.e., fish, chicken, etc) and a calorie target is specified. For example Day 7 of the 1500 Calorie diet specifies a chicken dinner and allows you 630 Calories.

First, you need to choose a restaurant where you have a fighting chance to achieve your calorie goal. Next, order simple, such as broiled chicken breast with steamed vegetables and brown rice. Tell the waiter you want no sauce, no gravy, nothing added. Then, knowing your calorie objective, and that most fish and chicken are about 50 Calories per ounce, most steamed vegetable servings average about 50 Calories per cup, and rice is about 100 Calories per ½ cup, decide how much to eat – and take the remainder home. If fresh fruit is not an option, pass on dessert and have the evening snack specified in the meal plan for that day.

Mediterranean Diet Info

As mentioned previously, the 1200 Calorie 90-Day Diet starts on page 17. There is a detailed meal plan for each of the 90 days. Associated with each day is a "Recipe of the Day" and a "Diet Tip of the Day."

After you complete the 90th day on the diet, if you still want to lose more weight a good alternative is to repeat the diet by starting over at Day 1.

Important Notes

1) Coffee may be decaf or regular. If desired, skim milk and a sugar substitute may be added to coffee or tea. And soy or almond milk may be used instead of cow's milk.

2) Fried eggs or scrambled eggs should be cooked in a pan coated with a non-stick cooking spray (see page 11). Hard-boiled eggs may be substituted for fried, scrambled or soft-boiled eggs.

3) Cereals should be whole grain and unsweetened. At the top of the list are Old-fashioned Oatmeal, Wheatena and Shredded Wheat. Among other reasonably healthy choices are Cheerios, Wheat Chex, Wheaties, some Kashi cereals and Farina. When blueberries are in season, you may add blueberries instead of raisins to your cereal. (Substitution ratio = 2 blueberries per raisin.)

4) Bread may be either plain or toasted whole grain, such as whole wheat, whole rye or pumpernickel. Look for whole grain varieties that contain 70 Calories per slice. If desired, bread may be topped with a home-made low-calorie olive oil spray. NO BUTTER!

5) When soup is specified, have only one serving (8 ounces) unless otherwise noted. (Most caned soups usually contain about two servings.)

6) Use freely as desired: clear unsweetened coffee, clear unsweetened tea, water, seltzer water and any diet soda, clear soups without fat, bouillon, and seasonings such as mustard, cinnamon, dill, herbs, red and black pepper, curry, vinegar, and lemon juice and lemon sections.

7) Use only lean cuts of meat trimmed of all visible fat. Poultry should be limited to chicken or turkey breasts (white meat only and skinless).

8) When canned tuna or salmon is specified, use only fish packed in water.

9) When the diet calls for turkey bacon, make sure the brand you buy has no more than 35 Calories per slice.

10) An unlimited amount of salad may be eaten, but the salad dressing should be as specified on page 11.

11) Use freely as desired: clear unsweetened coffee, clear unsweetened tea, water, seltzer, any diet soda, clear soups without fat, bouillon, and seasonings such as mustard, cinnamon, dill, herbs, red and black pepper, curry, vinegar, lemon juice and sections, and dill and sour pickles.

12) If it's more convenient, any food item may be moved to any part of the day and combined with any meal or snack.

13) If you cannot find the exact item called for in the diet (because it's out of stock or discontinued), substitute a comparable food (of the same type and close caloric value).

14) Although it's recommended that you follow the diet days as outlined, it's fine to occasionally pick and choose the days you prefer. (

1500 CALORIE DAILY MENUS

Day 1 – 1500 Calorie Meal Plan

BREAKFAST	Calories	Totals
Grapefruit (½)	75	
Scramble 2 eggs (page 14)	160	
Whole-grain toast (1 slice) (page 11)	65	
Coffee (page 14)	10	310 Cal
SNACK		
Greek Yogurt (6 oz, nonfat, any flavor)*	90	
Coffee or tea	10	100 Cal
LUNCH		
Salad – 3 oz canned salmon, 1 tsp Evoo, onions & celery	200	
Lettuce & tomato wedges	20	
Italian or French bread (1 slice) (page 14)	80	
Water	0	300 Cal
SNACK		
Handful of unsalted mixed nuts	100	100 Cal
DINNER		
Chicken w Peppers & Onions (Day 1 Recipe p. 108)	250	
Sautéed red peppers with onions	70	
Green beans (steamed) & mashed cauliflower	45	
Large salad with 2 Tbsp dressing (page 10)	150	
Fresh fruit in season (apple, plum, etc)	70	
Water with lemon wedge	10	595 Cal
SNACK		
Fiber One Chocolate Fudge Brownie	90	
Coffee or tea	10	100 Cal
* Such as Dannon Lite & Fit. (Buy 32 oz container & use 6 oz.)		1505 Cal

Day 2 – 1500 Calorie Meal Plan

BREAKFAST	Calories	Totals
Fresh or frozen strawberries (½ cup)	25	
French toasted English Muffin (Day 2 Recipe p 109)	270	
Light syrup (2 Tbsp)	60	
Coffee	10	365 Cal
SNACK		
Greek Yogurt (6 oz, nonfat, any flavor)	90	90 Cal
LUNCH		
Salad (3 oz tuna, 1 tsp Evoo, onions & celery)	175	
Lettuce & tomato wedges	20	
Italian or French bread (1 slice) (page 14)	80	
Fresh fruit in season (apple, peach, etc)	70	
Hot or iced tea	10	355 Cal
SNACK		
Handful mixed unsalted nuts	100	100 Cal
DINNER		
Broiled veal chop (4 oz lean)	200	
Broccoli (½ cup steamed)	25	
Large salad with 2 Tbsp dressing (page 10)	150	
Glass wine (red or white) (4 oz)	100	395 Cal
SNACK		
Kashi TLC Crunchy Granola Bar*	180	
Coffee or tea	10	190 Cal
* If unavailable an equivalent dessert.		1495 Cal

Day 3 – 1500 Calorie Meal Plan

BREAKFAST	Calories	Totals
Orange juice (½ cup)	50	
Wheaties (¾ cup) + ½ cup skim milk + ½ banana	190	
Coffee	10	250 Cal
SNACK		
Fresh fruit in season (apple, peach, etc)	70	70 Cal
LUNCH		
Soup (Appendix C - page 205)*	150	
Turkey breast (1 oz) on 1 slice bread (½ sandwich)	105	
Lettuce & tomato slices	20	
Fresh fruit in season (apple, peach, etc)	70	
Hot or ice tea	10	355 Cal
* 30 calories added to account for flavor enhancement.		
SNACK		
Greek Yogurt (6 oz, nonfat, any flavor)	90	90 Cal
DINNER		
Baked Herb-Crusted Cod (Day 3 Recipe page 110)	230	
Spinach (½ cup) steamed with garlic & drizzled Evoo	100	
Asparagus (7 spear cooked & drained)	20	
Italian or French bread (1 slice)	80	
Glass wine (red or white) (4 oz)	100	
Water	0	530 Cal
SNACK		
Fiber One Chocolate Fudge Brownie*	90	
Coffee or tea	10	100 Cal
* If unavailable an equivalent dessert.		1500 Cal

Day 4 – 1500 Calorie Meal Plan

BREAKFAST	Calories	Totals
Grapefruit (½)	75	
Cheerios (1 cup) + ½ cup skim milk + about 15 raisins*	180	
Coffee	10	265 Cal
SNACK		
Coffee or tea	10	10 Cal
LUNCH		
Subway 6" (Roast Beef, Cheese + veggies)**	245	
Large salad with 2 Tbsp dressing (page 10)	150	
Water	0	395 Cal
** On 6" half wheat roll.		
SNACK		
Fresh fruit in season (peach, plum, etc)	70	70 Cal
DINNER		
Pasta and Veggies (Day 4 Recipe - page 111)	460	
Italian or French bread (1 slice)	80	
Fresh fruit in season (peach, plum, etc)	70	
Glass of wine (4 oz)	100	710 Cal
SNACK		
Coffee or tea	10	10 Cal
* See page 14 re substituting blueberries for raisins.		1490 Cal

Day 5 – 1500 Calorie Meal Plan

BREAKFAST	Calories	Totals
Cantaloupe (½ medium)	50	
Fried egg	80	
Toasted raisin bread (1 slice)	75	
Coffee	10	215 Cal
SNACK		
Greek Yogurt (6 oz, nonfat, any flavor)	90	90 Cal
LUNCH		
Soup (Appendix C - page 205)	160	
Italian or French bread (1 slice)	80	
Lettuce and sliced tomato with 1 Tbsp dressing	85	
Hot or iced tea	10	335 Cal
* 30 calories added to account for flavor enhancement.		
SNACK		
Handful unsalted mixed nuts	100	100 Cal
DINNER		
Frozen fish dinner (Day 5 Recipe - page 112)	340	
Large salad with 2 Tbsp dressing	150	
Fresh fruit in season (apple, plum, etc)	70	
Glass of wine (4 oz)	100	660 Cal
SNACK		
One small cookie*	80	
Coffee or tea	10	90 Cal
* Oatmeal, ginger snap, sugar, etc - check calories!		1490 Cal

Day 6 – 1500 Calorie Meal Plan

BREAKFAST	Calories	Totals
Tomato juice (½ cup)	20	
Shredded Wheat (1 cup) + ½ cup skim milk + ½ banana	265	
Coffee	10	295 Cal
SNACK		
Coffee or tea	10	10 Cal
LUNCH		
Ham (2 oz) with mustard on 2 slices rye bread	290	
Lettuce	10	
Fresh fruit in season (pear, plum, etc)	70	
Water	0	360 Cal
SNACK		
Handful unsalted mixed nuts	100	100 Cal
DINNER		
Pizza (Day 6 Recipe - page 113)	350	
Large salad with 2 Tbsp dressing	150	
Glass of wine (4 oz)	100	600 Cal
SNACK		
Skinny Cow Ice Cream Sandwich*	160	160 Cal
* If unavailable an equivalent dessert.		1525 Cal

Day 7 – 1500 Calorie Meal Plan

BREAKFAST	Calories	Totals
Cantaloupe (½ medium)	50	
Oatmeal (½ cup dry) + ½ cup skim milk + about 15 raisins	220	
Coffee	10	280 Cal
SNACK		
Coffee or tea	10	10 Cal
LUNCH		
Grilled cheese sandwich (2 slices 2% cheese)	230	
Lettuce and sliced tomato	20	
Water	0	250 Cal
SNACK		
Handful of unsalted mixed nuts	100	
Coffee or tea	10	110 Cal
DINNER		
Eat Out – Chicken dinner (Day 7 Recipe - page 116)	530	
Glass wine (red or white) (4 oz)	100	630 Cal
SNACK		
Kashi TLC Crunchy Granola Bar	180	
Coffee or tea	10	190 Cal
		1480 Cal

Day 8 – 1500 Calorie Meal Plan

BREAKFAST	Calories	Totals
Cantaloupe (½ medium)	50	
Wheaties (¾ cup) + ½ cup skim milk + ½ banana	190	
Coffee	10	250 Cal
SNACK		
Fresh fruit in season (apple, plum, etc)	70	70 Cal
LUNCH		
Soup (Appendix C - page 205)*	120	
Turkey (1 oz) on 1 slice of rye bread (½ sandwich)	115	
Lettuce & tomato slices	20	
Hot or iced tea	10	265 Cal
* 30 calories added to account for flavor enhancement.		
SNACK		
Handful unsalted mixed nuts	100	100 Cal
DINNER		
Baked salmon with salsa (Day 8 Recipe - page 115)	215	
Summer squash, zucchini and tomatoes	60	
Brown rice (½ cup)	100	
Large salad with 2 Tbsp dressing	150	
Glass of wine (4 oz)	100	625 Cal
SNACK		
Kashi TLC Crunchy Granola Bar	180	
Coffee or tea	10	190 Cal
		1500 Cal

Day 9 – 1500 Calorie Meal Plan

BREAKFAST	Calories	Totals
Orange juice (½ cup)	50	
Soft-boiled egg	80	
Whole-grain toast (1 slice)	65	
Coffee	10	205 Cal
SNACK		
Coffee or tea	10	10 Cal
LUNCH		
Salad (3 oz tuna, 1 tsp Evoo, onions & celery)	175	
Lettuce & tomato wedges	20	
Rye bread (1 slice)	65	
Fresh fruit in season (pear, peach, etc)	70	
Water or diet soda	0	330 Cal
SNACK		
Greek Yogurt (6 oz, nonfat, any flavor)	90	
Coffee or tea	10	100 Cal
DINNER		
Veggie burger – (1 patty) (Day 9 Recipe - page 116)	100	
Low-fat cheddar cheese (1 thin slice)	50	
Seeded hamburger roll + Beets (3 small)	185	
Large salad with 2 Tbsp dressing	150	
Glass of wine (4 oz)	100	575 Cal
SNACK		
Fiber One Chocolate-Fudge Brownie	90	
Coffee or tea	10	100 Cal
		1490 Cal

Day 10 – 1500 Calorie Meal Plan

BREAKFAST	Calories	Totals
Orange juice (½ cup)	50	
Wild blueberry pancakes (Day 10 Recipe - page 117)	190	
Light syrup (2 Tbsp)	60	
Coffee	10	310 Cal
SNACK		
Greek Yogurt (6 oz, nonfat, any flavor)	90	90 Cal
LUNCH		
Peanut butter (2 Tbsp) on 2 slices whole-grain bread	330	
Skim milk (4 oz)	45	
Fresh fruit in season (apple, plum, etc)	70	445 Cal
SNACK		
Coffee or tea	10	10 Cal
DINNER		
Broiled pork chop (about ½" thick & trimmed of fat)	260	
Green peas (½ cup)	55	
Tomato & cucumbers salad with 1 Tbsp dressing	105	
Glass of wine (4 oz)	100	520Cal
SNACK		
Coffee or tea	10	10 Cal
		1485 Cal

Day 11 – 1500 Calorie Meal Plan

BREAKFAST	Calories	Totals
Fresh sliced orange	75	
Cheerios (1 cup) + ½ cup skim milk + about 15 raisins	190	
Coffee	10	275 Cal
SNACK		
Fresh fruit in season (apple, plum, etc)	70	70 Cal
LUNCH		
Subway 6" (Ham, Cheese + veggies)	260	
Water or diet soda	0	260 Cal
SNACK		
Handful unsalted mixed nuts	100	
Coffee or tea	10	110 Cal
DINNER		
Grilled chicken sausage (2 links about 2½ oz per link)	180	
Artichoke-bean salad (Day 11 Recipe - page 118)	190	
Green beans - steamed	25	
Italian or French bread (1 slice)	80	
Glass of wine (4 oz)	100	575 Cal
SNACK		
Kashi TLC Crunchy Granola Bar	180	
Coffee or tea	10	190 Cal
		1480 Cal

Day 12 – 1500 Calorie Meal Plan

BREAKFAST	Calories	Totals
Grapefruit (½)	75	
Scrambled egg	80	
Whole-grain toast (1 slice)	65	
Coffee	10	230 Cal
SNACK		
Greek Yogurt (6 oz, nonfat, any flavor)	90	90 Cal
LUNCH		
Soup (Appendix C - page 205)	140	
Tomato slices, ¼ cup chopped fresh basil + ½ tsp Evoo	40	
Whole-grain bread (1 slice)	65	
Hot or iced tea	10	265 Cal
* 30 calories added to account for flavor enhancement.		
SNACK		
Handful of unsalted mixed nuts	100	
Coffee or tea	10	110 Cal
DINNER		
Eat Out – Fish dinner (Day 12 Recipe page 119)	530	
Glass of wine (4 oz)	100	630 Cal
SNACK		
Fiber One Chocolate-Fudge Brownie	90	
Coffee or tea	10	100 Cal
* If unavailable an equivalent dessert.		1490 Cal

Day 13 – 1500 Calorie Meal Plan

BREAKFAST	Calories	Totals
Orange juice (½ cup)	50	
Shredded Wheat (1 cup) + ½ cup skim milk + ½ banana	260	
Coffee	10	320 Cal
SNACK		
Fresh fruit in season (pear, plum, etc)	70	70 Cal
LUNCH		
Turkey frank (2 oz) with mustard & relish	150	
Hot dog bun	125	
Water or diet soda	0	275 Cal
SNACK		
Greek Yogurt (6 oz, nonfat, any flavor)	90	90 Cal
DINNER		
Pasta with Marinara sauce (Day 13 Recipe - p. 120)	225	
Large salad with 2 Tbsp dressing	150	
Italian or French bread (1 slice)	80	
Glass of wine (4 oz)	100	555 Cal
SNACK		
Kashi TLC Crunchy Granola Bar	180	
Coffee or tea	10	190 Cal
		1500 Cal

Day 14 – 1500 Calorie Meal Plan

BREAKFAST	Calories	Totals
Cantaloupe (½ medium)	50	
Oatena cereal mix (Day 14 Recipe - page 121)	310	
Coffee	10	370 Cal
SNACK		
Fresh fruit in season (apple, peach, plum, etc)	70	70 Cal
LUNCH		
Grilled Swiss cheese sandwich (2 oz low-fat cheese)	310	
Diet soda or water	0	310 Cal
SNACK		
Large salad with 2 Tbsp dressing	100	
Coffee or tea	10	110 Cal
DINNER		
Frozen chicken dinner (Day 28 Recipe - page 135)	300	
Small salad with 1 Tbsp dressing	75	
Water	0	375 Cal
SNACK		
Greek Yogurt (6 oz, nonfat, any flavor)	90	90 Cal
		1500 Cal

Day 15 – 1500 Calorie Meal Plan

BREAKFAST	Calories	Totals
Fresh or frozen strawberries (1 cup)	50	
French toast (2 slices whole-grain bread & 1 egg)	250	
Light syrup (2 Tbsp)	60	
Coffee	10	370 Cal
SNACK		
Greek Yogurt (6 oz, nonfat, any flavor)	90	90 Cal
LUNCH		
Salad (3 oz tuna, 1 tsp Evoo, onions & celery)	175	
Lettuce & tomato wedges	20	
Rye bread (1 slice)	65	
Hot or iced tea	10	270 Cal
SNACK		
Handful unsalted mixed nuts	100	
Coffee or tea	10	110 Cal
DINNER		
London broil (Day 15 Recipe - page 122)	320	
Brown rice (½ cup)	100	
Broccoli (1 cup steamed)	50	
Glass of wine (4 oz)	100	570 Cal
SNACK		
Nature Valley Crunchy Granola Bar*	95	95 Cal
* If unavailable an equivalent dessert.		1505 Cal

Day 16 – 1500 Calorie Meal Plan

BREAKFAST	Calories	Totals
Orange juice (½ cup)	50	
Wheat Chex (¾ cup) + ½ cup skim milk + ½ banana	250	
Coffee	10	310 Cal
SNACK		
Fresh fruit in season (apple, peach, etc)	70	70 Cal
LUNCH		
Subway 6" (Roast Beef, Cheese + veggies)	245	
Diet soda or water	0	245 Cal
SNACK		
Handful unsalted mixed nuts	100	100 Cal
DINNER		
Baked red snapper (Day 16 Recipe - page 123)	215	
Wild rice mix	160	
Green beans & tomato	75	
Italian or French bread (1 slice)	80	
Glass of wine (4 oz)	100	630 Cal
SNACK		
Skinny Cow Ice Cream Sandwich	160	160 Cal
		1515 Cal

Day 17 – 1500 Calorie Meal Plan

BREAKFAST	Calories	Totals
Cantaloupe (½ medium)	50	
Fried egg	80	
Turkey bacon (1 slice)	35	
Toasted raisin bread (2 slices)	150	
Coffee	10	325 Cal
SNACK		
Greek Yogurt (6 oz, nonfat, any flavor)	90	90 Cal
LUNCH		
Soup (Appendix C - page 205)	160	
Lettuce & tomato sandwich with Tbsp light mayo	170	
Cucumber slices and carrot & celery sticks	15	
Water	0	345 Cal
SNACK		
Fresh fruit in season (apple, peach, plum, etc)	70	70 Cal
DINNER		
Cajun chicken salad (Day 17 Recipe - page 124)	330	
Whole-grain bread (1 slice)	65	
Fresh fruit in season (pear, plum, etc)	70	
Glass of wine (4 oz)	100	565 Cal
SNACK		
Kashi TLC Crunchy Granola Bar	180	180 Cal
		1525 Cal

Day 18 – 1500 Calorie Meal Plan

BREAKFAST	Calories	Totals
Grapefruit (½)	75	
Cheerios (1 cup) + ½ cup skim milk + about 15 raisins	190	
Coffee	10	275 Cal
SNACK		
Fresh fruit in season (peach, plum, etc)	70	70 Cal
LUNCH		
Cottage cheese (1 cup low fat)	180	
Small salad with 1 Tbsp low-cal dressing (page 10)	75	
Hot or iced tea	10	265 Cal
SNACK		
Handful unsalted mixed nuts	100	
Coffee or tea	10	110 Cal
DINNER		
Grilled swordfish (Day 18 Recipe - page 125)	250	
Grilled potatoes	100	
Grilled cherry tomatoes	40	
Spinach (½ cup) steamed with garlic & drizzled Evoo	50	
Glass of wine (4 oz)	100	540 Cal
SNACK		
Fiber One Chocolate Fudge Brownie	90	
Coffee or tea	10	100 Cal
		1480 Cal

Day 19 – 1500 Calorie Meal Plan

BREAKFAST	Calories	Totals
Grapefruit (½)	75	
Scrambled egg	80	
Whole-grain toast (2 slices)	130	
Coffee	10	295 Cal
SNACK		
Greek Yogurt (6 oz, nonfat, any flavor)	90	90 Cal
LUNCH		
Soup (Appendix C - page 205)	180	
Turkey (1 oz) on 1 slice of rye bread (½ sandwich)	115	
Hot or iced tea	10	305 Cal
SNACK		
Coffee or tea	10	10 Cal
DINNER		
Eat Out – Italian food (Day 19 Recipe - page 126)	530	
Glass of wine (4 oz)	100	630 Cal
SNACK		
Skinny Cow Ice Cream Sandwich	160	160 Cal
		1500 Cal

Day 20 – 1500 Calorie Meal Plan

BREAKFAST	Calories	Totals
Tomato juice (½ cup)	20	
Shredded Wheat (1 cup) + ½ cup skim milk	210	
Coffee	10	240 Cal
SNACK		
Handful unsalted mixed nuts	100	100 Cal
LUNCH		
Left over Italian food from Day 19	260	
Hot or iced tea	10	270 Cal
SNACK		
Fresh fruit in season (apple, peach, plum, etc)	70	70 Cal
DINNER		
Spaghetti alla Puttanesca (Day 20 Recipe - page 127)	345	
Large salad with 2 Tbsp dressing	150	
Italian or French bread (1 slice)	80	
Glass of wine (4 oz)	100	675 Cal
SNACK		
Skinny Cow Ice Cream Sandwich	160	160 Cal
		1515 Cal

Day 21 – 1500 Calorie Meal Plan

BREAKFAST	Calories	Totals
Cantaloupe (½ medium)	50	
Oatmeal (½ cup dry) + ½ cup skim milk + about 15 raisins	220	
Coffee	10	280 Cal
SNACK		
Handful unsalted mixed nuts	100	
Coffee or tea	10	110 Cal
LUNCH		
Turkey breast (2 oz) sandwich	235	
Lettuce & tomato with Tbsp light mayo	35	
Fresh fruit in season (apple, plum, etc)	70	
Water	0	340 Cal
SNACK		
Coffee or tea	10	10 Cal
DINNER		
Frozen meat dinner (Day 21 Recipe - page 128)	300	
Large salad with 2 Tbsp dressing	150	
Italian or French bread (1 slice)	80	
Glass of wine (4 oz)	100	630 Cal
SNACK		
Graham crackers (4 squares)	120	
Coffee or tea	10	130 Cal
		1500 Cal

Day 22 – 1500 Calorie Meal Plan

BREAKFAST	Calories	Totals
Fresh or frozen strawberries (1 cup)	25	
French toasted English Muffin (Day 2 Recipe p.109)	270	
Light syrup (2 Tbsp)	60	
Coffee	10	365 Cal
SNACK		
Greek Yogurt (6 oz, nonfat, any flavor)	90	90 Cal
LUNCH		
Salad (3 oz tuna, 1 tsp Evoo, onions & celery)	175	
Lettuce & tomato wedges	20	
Fresh fruit in season (apple, peach, plum, etc)	70	
Hot or iced tea	10	275 Cal
SNACK		
Handful unsalted mixed nuts	100	
Coffee or tea	10	110 Cal
DINNER		
Shrimp & spinach salad (Day 22 Recipe - page 129)	310	
Italian or French bread (1 slice)	80	
Large salad with 2 Tbsp dressing	150	
Glass of wine (4 oz)	100	640 Cal
SNACK		
Coffee or tea	10	10 Cal
		1490 Cal

Day 23 – 1500 Calorie Meal Plan

BREAKFAST	Calories	Totals
Cantaloupe (½ medium)	50	
Wheaties (¾ cup) + ½ cup skim milk + ½ banana	190	
Whole-grain toast (1 slice)	65	
Coffee	10	315 Cal
SNACK		
Fresh fruit in season (apple, peach, etc)	70	70 Cal
LUNCH		
Ham (2 oz) with mustard on 2 slices rye bread	290	
Lettuce & tomato wedges	20	
Water or diet soda	0	310 Cal
SNACK		
Handful unsalted mixed nuts	100	
Coffee or tea	10	110 Cal
DINNER		
Beans & greens salad (Day 23 Recipe - page 130)	260	
Baked potato (medium)	100	
Italian or French bread (1 slice)	80	
Glass of wine (4 oz)	100	540 Cal
SNACK		
Skinny Cow Ice Cream Sandwich	160	160 Cal
		1505 Cal

Day 24 – 1500 Calorie Meal Plan

BREAKFAST	Calories	Totals
Fresh orange sliced	75	
Soft-boiled egg	80	
Whole-grain toast (2 slices)	130	
Coffee	10	295 Cal
SNACK		
Greek Yogurt (6 oz, nonfat, any flavor)	90	90 Cal
LUNCH		
Salad – 3 oz salmon, 1 tsp Evoo, onions & celery	200	
Lettuce & tomato wedges	20	
Italian or French bread (1 slice)	80	
Coffee or tea	10	310 Cal
SNACK		
Handful unsalted mixed nuts	100	100 Cal
DINNER		
Chicken breast – broiled (5 oz)	240	
Four bean plus salad (½ cup) (Day 24 Recipe p 131)	135	
Large salad with 2 Tbsp dressing	150	
Glass of wine (4 oz)	100	625 Cal
SNACK		
Fresh fruit in season (pear, plum, etc)	70	70 Cal
		1500 Cal

Day 25 – 1500 Calorie Meal Plan

BREAKFAST	Calories	Totals
Grapefruit (½)	75	
Cheerios (1 cup) + ½ cup skim milk + about 15 raisins	190	
Coffee	10	275 Cal
SNACK		
Fresh fruit in season (peach, plum, etc)	70	70 Cal
LUNCH		
Subway 6" (Ham, Cheese + veggies)	260	
Diet soda or water	0	260 Cal
SNACK		
Handful unsalted mixed nuts	100	
Coffee or tea	10	110 Cal
DINNER		
Hanger steak (Day 25 Recipe - page 132)	320	
Roasted potatoes (Day 25 Recipe)	120	
Cherry tomatoes (Day 25 Recipe)	20	
Steamed spinach (½ cup)	25	
Italian or French bread (1 slice)	80	
Glass of wine (4 oz)	100	665 Cal
SNACK		
Graham crackers (4 squares)	120	
Coffee or tea	10	130 Cal
		1510 Cal

Day 26 – 1500 Calorie Meal Plan

BREAKFAST	Calories	Totals
Cantaloupe (½ medium)	50	
Fried egg	80	
Toasted whole-grain bread (2 slice2)	130	
Coffee	10	270 Cal
SNACK		
Greek Yogurt (6 oz, nonfat, any flavor)	90	90 Cal
LUNCH		
Soup (Appendix C - page 205)	200	
Italian or French bread (1 slice)	80	
Lettuce & tomato slices	20	
Fresh fruit in season (apple, plum, etc)	70	
Hot or iced tea	10	380 Cal
SNACK		
Handful unsalted mixed nuts	100	100 Cal
DINNER		
Grilled scallops (Day 26 Recipe - page 133)	210	
Grilled polenta (Day 26 Recipe)	125	
Mushroom-steamed green beans-red onion	45	
Grilled asparagus	10	
Glass of wine (4 oz)	100	490 Cal
SNACK		
Kashi TLC Crunchy Granola Bar	180	180 Cal
		1510 Cal

Day 27 – 1500 Calorie Meal Plan

BREAKFAST	Calories	Totals
Cantaloupe (½ medium)	50	
Oatmeal (½ cup dry) + ½ cup skim milk + 15 raisins	220	
Coffee	10	280 Cal
SNACK		
Fresh fruit in season (pear, plum, etc)	70	70 Cal
LUNCH		
Two servings (1 cup) left over Day 24 bean salad	270	
Italian or French bread (1 slice)	80	
Lettuce & tomato slices	20	
Water	0	370 Cal
SNACK		
Coffee or tea	10	10 Cal
DINNER		
Fettuccine (Day 27 Recipe - page 134)	290	
Large salad with 2 Tbsp dressing	150	
Italian or French bread (1 slice)	80	
Glass of wine (4 oz)	100	620 Cal
SNACK		
Skinny Cow Ice Cream Sandwich	160	160 Cal
		1510 Cal

Day 28 – 1500 Calorie Meal Plan

BREAKFAST	Calories	Totals
Tomato juice (½ cup)	20	
Shredded Wheat (1 cup) + ½ cup skim milk + ½ banana	260	
Coffee	10	290 Cal
SNACK		
Coffee or tea	10	10 Cal
LUNCH		
Roast beef sandwich (2 oz) on whole-grain bread	295	
Lettuce	0	
Fresh fruit in season (peach, plum, etc)	70	
Hot or iced tea	10	375 Cal
SNACK		
Handful unsalted mixed nuts	100	
Coffee or tea	10	110 Cal
DINNER		
Frozen chicken dinner (**Day 28 Recipe -** page 135)	300	
Large salad with 2 Tbsp dressing	150	
Italian or French bread (1 slice)	80	
Glass of wine (4 oz)	100	515 Cal
SNACK		
Kashi TLC Crunchy Granola Bar	180	
Coffee or tea	10	190 Cal
		1490 Cal

Day 29 – 1500 Calorie Meal Plan

BREAKFAST	Calories	Totals
Orange juice (½ cup)	50	
Wild blueberry pancakes (Day 10 Recipe - page 117)	190	
Turkey bacon (1 slice)	35	
Light syrup (2 Tbsp)	60	
Coffee	10	345 Cal
SNACK		
Greek Yogurt (6 oz, nonfat, any flavor)	90	90 Cal
LUNCH		
Salad (3 oz tuna, 1 tsp Evoo, onions & celery)	175	
Lettuce & tomato wedges	20	
Italian or French bread	80	
Hot or ice tea	10	285 Cal
SNACK		
Handful unsalted mixed nuts	100	
Coffee or tea	10	110 Cal
DINNER		
Barbequed shrimp (Day 29 Recipe - page 136)	160	
Corn on the cob (medium)	100	
Steamed broccoli (1 cup equivalent)	50	
Fresh fruit in season (apple, peach, etc)	70	
Glass of wine (4 oz)	100	480 Cal
SNACK		
Kashi TLC Crunchy Granola Bar	180	
Coffee or tea	10	190 Cal
		1500 Cal

Day 30 – 1500 Calorie Meal Plan

BREAKFAST	Calories	Totals
Fresh orange sliced	75	
Wheat Chex (¾ cup) + ½ cup skim milk + ½ banana	250	
Coffee	10	335 Cal
SNACK		
Coffee or tea	10	10 Cal
LUNCH		
Soup (Appendix C - page 205)	170	
Italian or French bread (1 slice)	80	
Fresh fruit in season (apple, peach, etc)	70	
Hot or iced tea	10	330 Cal
SNACK		
Handful unsalted mixed nuts	100	
Coffee or tea	10	110 Cal
DINNER		
Pasta e Fagioli (Day 30 Recipe - page 137)	300	
Small salad with 1 Tbsp dressing	75	
Italian or French bread (1 slice)	80	
Glass of wine (4 oz)	100	555 Cal
SNACK		
Skinny Cow Ice Cream Sandwich	160	160 Cal
		1500 Cal

Day 31 – 1500 Calorie Meal Plan

BREAKFAST	Calories	Totals
Tomato juice (½ cup)	20	
Wheaties (¾ cup) + ½ cup skim milk + ½ banana	190	
Coffee	10	220 Cal
SNACK		
Coffee or tea	10	10 Cal
LUNCH		
Ham (2 oz) with mustard on 2 slices rye bread	300	
Fresh fruit in season (apple, plum, etc)	70	
Diet soda or water	0	370 Cal
SNACK		
Handful unsalted mixed nuts	100	
Coffee or tea	10	110 Cal
DINNER		
Baked Sea Bass (Day 31 Recipe - page 138)	395	
Large salad with 2 Tbsp dressing	150	
Italian or French bread (1 slice)	80	
Glass of wine (4 oz)	100	725 Cal
SNACK		
Graham crackers (2 squares)	60	
Coffee or tea	10	70 Cal
		1505 Cal

Day 32 – 1500 Calorie Meal Plan

BREAKFAST	Calories	Totals
Tomato juice (½ cup)	20	
Cheerios (1 cup) + ½ cup skim milk + about 15 raisins	190	
Coffee	10	220 Cal
SNACK		
Coffee or tea	10	10 Cal
LUNCH		
Soup (Appendix C - page 205)	120	
Italian or French bread (1 slice)	80	
Fresh fruit in season (apple, plum, etc)	70	
Water	0	270 Cal
SNACK		
Handful unsalted mixed nuts	100	
Coffee or tea	10	110 Cal
DINNER		
Turkey tenders & veggies (Day 32 Recipe - page 139)	350	
Spinach (½ cup steamed & drizzled w 1 tsp Evoo)	70	
Large salad with 2 Tbsp dressing	150	
Italian or French bread (1 slice)	80	
Glass of wine (4 oz)	100	760 Cal
SNACK		
Graham crackers (4 squares)	120	
Coffee or tea	10	130 Cal
		1500 Cal

Day 33 – 1500 Calorie Meal Plan

BREAKFAST	Calories	Totals
Cantaloupe (½ medium)	50	
Fried egg	80	
Toasted raisin bread (2 slices)	150	
Coffee	10	290 Cal
SNACK		
Greek Yogurt (6 oz, nonfat, any flavor)	90	90 Cal
LUNCH		
Subway 6" (Turkey Breast, Cheese + veggies)	230	
Fresh fruit in season (apple, plum, etc)	70	
Water	0	300 Cal
SNACK		
Coffee or tea	10	10 Cal
DINNER		
Frozen fish dinner (Day 33 Recipe - page 140)	340	
Large salad with 2 Tbsp dressing	150	
Italian or French bread (1 slice)	80	
Glass of wine (4 oz)	100	670 Cal
SNACK		
Graham crackers (4 squares)	120	
Coffee or tea	10	130 Cal
		1490 Cal

Day 34 – 1500 Calorie Meal Plan

BREAKFAST	Calories	Totals
Tomato juice (½ cup)	20	
Shredded Wheat (1 cup) + ½ cup skim milk + ½ banana	265	
Coffee	10	295 Cal
SNACK		
Coffee or tea	10	10 Cal
LUNCH		
Roast beef (2 oz) sandwich (with lettuce)	300	
Fresh fruit in season (apple, pear, etc)	70	
Hot or iced tea	10	380 Cal
SNACK		
Handful unsalted mixed nuts	100	100 Cal
DINNER		
Pasta Rapini (Day 34 Recipe - page 141)	290	
Large salad with 2 Tbsp dressing	150	
Italian or French bread (1 slice)	80	
Glass of wine (4 oz)	100	620 Cal
SNACK		
Fiber One Chocolate Fudge Brownie	90	
Coffee or tea	10	100 Cal
		1505 Cal

Day 35 – 1500 Calorie Meal Plan

BREAKFAST	Calories	Totals
Cantaloupe (½ medium)	50	
Oatmeal (½ cup dry) + ½ cup skim milk + 15 raisins	220	
Whole grain bread (1 slice)	65	
Coffee	10	345 Cal
SNACK		
Coffee or tea	10	10 Cal
LUNCH		
Grilled cheese sandwich (2 slices 2% cheese)	240	
Fresh fruit in season (apple, plum, etc)	70	
Diet soda or water	0	310 Cal
SNACK		
Handful unsalted mixed nuts	100	
Coffee or tea	10	110 Cal
DINNER		
Eat Out – Chicken dinner (Day 35 Recipe page 142)	530	
Glass of wine (4 oz)	100	630 Cal
SNACK		
Fiber One Chocolate Fudge Brownie	90	
Coffee or tea	10	100 Cal
		1505 Cal

Day 36 – 1500 Calorie Meal Plan

BREAKFAST	Calories	Totals
Cantaloupe (½ medium)	50	
Wheaties (¾ cup) + ½ cup skim milk + ½ banana	190	
Coffee	10	250 Cal
SNACK		
Fresh fruit in season (apple, pear, etc)	70	70 Cal
LUNCH		
Soup (Appendix C - page 205)	120	
Turkey (1 oz) on 1 slice of rye bread (½ sandwich)	120	
Hot or ice tea	10	250 Cal
SNACK		
Handful unsalted mixed nuts	100	
Coffee or tea	10	110 Cal
DINNER		
Grilled Tilapia (Day 36 Recipe - page 143)	300	
Asparagus spear (6)	25	
Wild rice (½ cup – after cooking)	100	
Small salad with 1 Tbsp dressing	75	
Italian or French bread (1 slice)	80	
Glass of wine (4 oz)	100	680 Cal
SNACK		
Skinny Cow Ice Cream Sandwich	160	160 Cal
		1520 Cal

Day 37 – 1500 Calorie Meal Plan

BREAKFAST	Calories	Totals
Orange juice (½ cup)	50	
Soft-boiled egg	80	
Whole grain toast (2 slices)	130	
Coffee	10	270 Cal
SNACK		
Greek Yogurt (6 oz, nonfat, any flavor)	90	
Coffee or tea	10	100 Cal
LUNCH		
Salad (3 oz canned tuna, 1 tsp Evoo, onions, celery)	175	
Lettuce & tomato wedges	20	
Italian or French bread (1 slice)	80	
Water	0	275 Cal
SNACK		
Fresh fruit in season (apple, plum, etc)	70	
Coffee or tea	10	90 Cal
DINNER		
Crab Cakes (Day 37 Recipe - page 144)	320	
Large salad with 2 Tbsp dressing	150	
Glass of wine (4 oz)	100	570 Cal
SNACK		
Kashi TLC Crunchy Granola Bar	180	
Coffee or tea	10	190 Cal
		1485 Cal

Day 38 – 1500 Calorie Meal Plan

BREAKFAST	Calories	Totals
Cantaloupe (½ medium)	50	
Fried egg	80	
Toasted raisin bread (2 slices)	150	
Coffee	10	290 Cal
SNACK		
Greek Yogurt (6 oz, nonfat, any flavor)	90	90 Cal
LUNCH		
Peanut butter (2 Tbsp) on 2 slices bread	340	
Skim milk (4 oz)	45	385 Cal
SNACK		
Fresh fruit in season (apple, peach, etc)	70	70 Cal
DINNER		
Pan-broiled lamb chop (Day 38 Recipe - page 145)	320	
Large salad with 2 Tbsp dressing	150	
Italian or French bread (1 slice)	80	
Glass of wine (4 oz)	100	650 Cal
SNACK		
Coffee or tea	10	10 Cal
		1495 Cal

Day 39 – 1500 Calorie Meal Plan

BREAKFAST	Calories	Totals
Fresh sliced orange	75	
Cheerios (1 cup) + ½ cup skim milk + about 15 raisins	190	
Coffee	10	275 Cal
SNACK		
Fresh fruit in season (apple, plum, etc)	70	70 Cal
LUNCH		
Cottage cheese (1 cup low fat)	180	
Small salad with 1 Tbsp dressing	75	
Italian or French bread (1 slice)	80	
Hot or iced tea	10	345 Cal
SNACK		
Handful unsalted mixed nuts	100	100 Cal
DINNER		
Chicken with veggies (Day 39 Recipe - page 146)	365	
Italian or French bread (1 slice)	80	
Glass of wine (4 oz)	100	545 Cal
SNACK		
Skinny Cow Ice Cream Sandwich	160	160 Cal
		1495 Cal

Day 40 – 1500 Calorie Meal Plan

BREAKFAST	Calories	Totals
Grapefruit (½)	75	
Scrambled egg	80	
Toasted raisin bread (2 slices)	150	
Coffee	10	315 Cal
SNACK		
Greek Yogurt (6 oz, nonfat, any flavor)	90	90 Cal
LUNCH		
Soup (Appendix C - page 205)	190	
Italian or French bread (1 slice)	80	
Hot or iced tea	10	280 Cal
SNACK		
Handful unsalted mixed nuts	100	
Coffee or tea	10	110 Cal
DINNER		
Eat Out – Fish dinner (Day 40 Recipe - page 147)	495	
Glass of wine (4 oz)	100	595 Cal
SNACK		
Fiber One Chocolate Fudge Brownie	90	
Coffee or tea	10	100 Cal
		1490 Cal

Day 41 – 1500 Calorie Meal Plan

BREAKFAST	Calories	Totals
Orange juice (½ cup)	50	
Shredded Wheat (1 cup) + ½ cup skim milk + ½ banana	260	
Coffee	10	320 Cal
SNACK		
Fresh fruit in season (apple, peach, etc)	70	70 Cal
LUNCH		
Turkey frank (2 oz) with mustard & relish	150	
Hot dog bun	130	
Diet soda or water	0	280 Cal
SNACK		
Small bunch of grapes	65	65 Cal
DINNER		
Tina's Frittata (Day 41 Recipe - page 148)	320	
Large salad with 2 Tbsp dressing	150	
Italian or French bread (1 slice)	80	
Glass of wine (4 oz)	100	650 Cal
SNACK		
Nature Valley Crunchy Granola Bar	95	
Coffee or tea	10	105 Cal
		1490 Cal

Day 42 – 1500 Calorie Meal Plan

BREAKFAST	Calories	Totals
Cantaloupe (½ medium)	50	
Wheaties (¾ cup) + ½ cup skim milk + ½ banana	190	
Whole grain toast (1 slice)	65	
Coffee	10	315 Cal
SNACK		
Coffee or tea	10	10 Cal
LUNCH		
Grilled Swiss cheese sandwich (2 oz low-fat cheese)	310	
Fresh fruit in season (apple, peach, etc)	70	
Hot or iced tea	10	390 Cal
SNACK		
Coffee or tea	10	10 Cal
DINNER		
Frozen chicken dinner (Day 28 Recipe - page 135)	300	
Large salad with 2 Tbsp dressing	150	
Italian or French bread (1 slice)	80	
Glass of wine (4 oz)	100	630 Cal
SNACK		
Blueberry Muffin (Day 42 Recipe - page 149)	145	
Coffee or tea	10	155 Cal
		1510 Cal

Day 43 – 1500 Calorie Meal Plan

BREAKFAST	Calories	Totals
Fresh or frozen strawberries (½ cup)	25	
Fried egg	80	
Toasted raisin bread (2 slices)	150	
Coffee	10	265 Cal
SNACK		
Greek Yogurt (6 oz, nonfat, any flavor)	90	90 Cal
LUNCH		
Salad (3 oz canned tuna, 1 tsp Evoo, onions, celery)	175	
Lettuce & tomato wedges	20	
Rye bread (1 slice)	70	
Fresh fruit in season (apple, plum, etc)	70	
Coffee or tea	10	345 Cal
SNACK		
Handful unsalted mixed nuts	100	100 Cal
DINNER		
Beef Kebob with veggies (Day 43 Recipe - page 150)	390	
Italian or French bread (1 slice)	80	
Glass of wine (4 oz)	100	570 Cal
SNACK		
Graham crackers (4 squares)	120	
Coffee or tea	10	130 Cal
		1500 Cal

Day 44 – 1500 Calorie Meal Plan

BREAKFAST	Calories	Totals
Orange juice (½ cup)	50	
Kashi GoLean (1 cup) + ½ cup skim milk + ½ banana	235	
Coffee	10	295 Cal
SNACK		
Handful unsalted mixed nuts	100	100 Cal
LUNCH		
Soup (Appendix C - page 205)	110	
Italian or French bread (1 slice)	80	
Fresh fruit in season (apple, plum, etc)	70	
Hot or iced tea	10	270 Cal
SNACK		
Nature Valley Crunchy Granola Bar	95	95 Cal
DINNER		
Baked Haddock (Day 44 Recipe - page 151)	420	
Large salad with 2 Tbsp dressing	150	
Italian or French bread (1 slice)	80	
Glass of wine (4 oz)	100	750 Cal
SNACK		
Coffee or tea	10	10 Cal
		1520 Cal

Day 45 – 1500 Calorie Meal Plan

BREAKFAST	Calories	Totals
Cantaloupe (½ medium)	50	
Scrambled egg	80	
Toasted whole-grain bread (2 slices)	130	
Coffee	10	270 Cal
SNACK		
Greek Yogurt (6 oz nonfat, any flavor)	90	90 Cal
LUNCH		
Soup (Appendix C - page 205)	190	
Lettuce & tomato sandwich (1 Tbsp light mayo)	170	
Water	0	360 Cal
SNACK		
Coffee or tea	10	10 Cal
DINNER		
Chicken Cacciatore (Day 45 Recipe - page 152)	310	
Large salad with 2 Tbsp dressing	150	
Italian or French bread (1 slice)	80	
Glass of wine (4 oz)	100	640 Cal
SNACK		
Blueberry muffin	145	
Coffee or tea	10	155 Cal
		1525 Cal

Day 46 – 1500 Calorie Meal Plan

BREAKFAST	Calories	Totals
Grapefruit (½)	75	
Cheerios (1 cup) + ½ cup skim milk + about 15 raisins	190	
Coffee	10	275 Cal
SNACK		
Fresh fruit in season (apple, peach, etc)	70	70 Cal
LUNCH		
Subway 6" (Ham, Cheese + veggies)	260	
Diet soda or water	0	260 Cal
SNACK		
Handful unsalted mixed nuts	100	100 Cal
DINNER		
Poached Cod (Day 46 Recipe - page 153)	275	
Grilled potatoes	100	
Grilled cherry tomatoes	45	
Spinach (½ cup) steamed with garlic & drizzled	50	
Italian or French bread (1 slice)	80	
Glass of wine (4 oz)	100	650 Cal
SNACK		
Blueberry muffin	145	
Coffee or tea	10	155 Cal
		1520 Cal

Day 47 – 1500 Calorie Meal Plan

BREAKFAST	Calories	Totals
Grapefruit (½)	75	
Fried egg	80	
Whole-grain toast (2 slices)	130	
Coffee	10	295 Cal
SNACK		
Fresh fruit in season (apple, plum, etc)	70	70 Cal
LUNCH		
Salad (3 oz canned tuna, 1 tsp Evoo, onions, celery)	175	
Lettuce & tomato wedges	20	
Rye bread (1 slice)	70	
Coffee or tea	10	275 Cal
SNACK		
Handful unsalted mixed nuts	100	100 Cal
DINNER		
Black-eyed peas &Rice (Day 47 Recipe - page 154)	280	
Large salad with 2 Tbsp dressing	150	
Italian or French bread (1 slice)	80	
Glass of wine (4 oz)	100	610 Cal
SNACK		
Blueberry muffin	145	
Coffee or tea	10	155 Cal
		1505 Cal

Day 48 – 1500 Calorie Meal Plan

BREAKFAST	Calories	Totals
Cantaloupe (½ medium)	50	
Oatena cereal mix (Day 14 Recipe - page 121)	310	
Coffee	10	370 Cal
SNACK		
Fresh fruit in season (apple, peach, etc)	70	70 Cal
LUNCH		
Subway 6" (Ham, Cheese + veggies)	260	
Diet soda or water	0	260 Cal
SNACK		
Coffee or tea	10	10 Cal
DINNER		
Pasta Salad (Day 48 Recipe - page 155)	370	
Large salad with 2 Tbsp dressing	150	
Italian or French bread (1 slice)	80	
Glass of wine (4 oz)	100	700 Cal
SNACK		
Graham crackers (2 squares)	60	
Coffee or tea	10	70 Cal
		1480 Cal

Day 49 – 1500 Calorie Meal Plan

BREAKFAST	Calories	Totals
Cantaloupe (½ medium)	50	
Oatmeal (½ cup dry) + ½ cup skim milk + about 15 raisins	220	
Coffee	10	280 Cal
SNACK		
Greek Yogurt (6 oz nonfat, any flavor)	90	90 Cal
LUNCH		
Turkey breast (2 oz) on 2 slices whole-grain bread	245	
Lettuce, tomato and 1 Tbsp light mayo	35	
Water with lemon wedge	10	290 Cal
SNACK		
Fresh fruit in season (apple, peach, etc)	70	70 Cal
DINNER		
Frozen meat dinner (Day 49 Recipe - page 156)	300	
Large salad with 2 Tbsp dressing	150	
Italian or French bread (1 slice)	80	
Glass of wine (4 oz)	100	630 Cal
SNACK		
Blueberry muffin	145	
Coffee or tea	10	155 Cal
		1515 Cal

Day 50 – 1500 Calorie Meal Plan

BREAKFAST	Calories	Totals
Fresh or frozen strawberries (1 cup)	25	
French toasted English Muffin (Day 2 Recipe p 109)	270	
Light syrup (2 Tbsp)	60	
Coffee	10	365 Cal
SNACK		
Greek Yogurt (6 oz nonfat, any flavor)	90	90 Cal
LUNCH		
Soup (Appendix C - page 205)	110	
BLT sandwich (2 slices turkey bacon, 1 Tbsp light mayo)	245	
Fresh fruit in season (apple, peach, etc)	70	
Hot or iced tea	10	435 Cal
SNACK		
Coffee or tea	10	10 Cal
DINNER		
Pan-fried Sole (Day 50 Recipe - page 157)	325	
Small salad with 1 Tbsp dressing	75	
Italian or French bread (1 slice)	80	
Glass of wine (4 oz)	100	580 Cal
SNACK		
Coffee or tea	10	10 Cal
		1490 Cal

Day 51 – 1500 Calorie Meal Plan

BREAKFAST	Calories	Totals
Cantaloupe (½ medium)	50	
Wheaties (¾ cup) + ½ cup skim milk + ½ banana	190	
Coffee	10	250 Cal
SNACK		
Toasted raisin bread (1 slice)	75	
Coffee or tea	10	85 Cal
LUNCH		
Ham (2 oz) with mustard on 2 slices rye bread	290	
Fresh fruit in season (pear, peach, etc)	70	
Hot or iced tea	10	370 Cal
SNACK		
Handful unsalted mixed nuts	100	
Coffee or tea	10	110 Cal
DINNER		
Beans and Greens Salad (Day 51 Recipe - page 158)	260	
Baked potato (medium)	100	
Italian or French bread (1 slice)	80	
Glass of wine (4 oz)	100	540 Cal
SNACK		
Graham crackers (4 squares)	120	
Coffee or tea	10	130 Cal
		1485 Cal

Day 52 – 1500 Calorie Meal Plan

BREAKFAST	Calories	Totals
Fresh orange sliced	75	
Soft-boiled egg	80	
Whole-grain toast (2 slices)	140	
Coffee	10	305 Cal
SNACK		
Greek Yogurt (6 oz nonfat, any flavor)	90	90 Cal
LUNCH		
Salad – 3 oz canned salmon, 1 tsp Evoo, onions & celery	200	
Lettuce & tomato wedges	20	
Italian or French bread (1 slice)	70	
Fresh fruit in season (apple, plum, etc)	70	
Hot or iced tea	10	370 Cal
SNACK		
Handful unsalted mixed nuts	100	
Coffee or tea	10	110 Cal
DINNER		
Chicken Piccata (Day 52 Recipe - page 159)	270	
Brown rice (½ cup – after cooking)	100	
Large salad with 2 Tbsp dressing	150	
Glass of wine (4 oz)	100	615 Cal
SNACK		
Coffee or tea	10	10 Cal
		1500 Cal

Day 53 – 1500 Calorie Meal Plan

BREAKFAST	Calories	Totals
Grapefruit (½)	75	
Cheerios (1 cup) + ½ cup skim milk + about 15 raisins	190	
Coffee	10	275 Cal
SNACK		
Fresh fruit in season (peach, plum, etc)	70	
Coffee or tea	10	80 Cal
LUNCH		
Cottage cheese (1 cup low fat)	180	
Large salad with 2 Tbsp dressing	150	
Hot or iced tea	10	340 Cal
SNACK		
Coffee or tea	10	10 Cal
DINNER		
Pasta Primavera (Day 53 Recipe - page 160)	350	
Small salad with 1 Tbsp dressing	75	
Italian or French bread (1 slice)	80	
Glass of wine (4 oz)	100	605 Cal
SNACK		
Kashi TLC Crunchy Granola Bar	180	
Coffee or tea	10	190 Cal
		1500 Cal

Day 54 – 1500 Calorie Meal Plan

BREAKFAST	Calories	Totals
Cantaloupe (½ medium)	50	
Fried egg	80	
Toasted whole-grain bread (2 slices)	130	
Coffee	10	270 Cal
SNACK		
Greek Yogurt (6 oz nonfat, any flavor)	90	90 Cal
LUNCH		
Soup (Appendix C - page 205)	200	
Italian or French bread (1 slice)	80	
Fresh fruit in season (plum, peach, etc)	70	
Water	0	350 Cal
SNACK		
Handful unsalted mixed nuts	100	100 Cal
DINNER		
Grilled scallops (Day 54 Recipe - page 161)	210	
Grilled polenta (Day 54 Recipe)	125	
Mushroom-steamed green beans-red onion (Day 54	45	
Grilled asparagus (Day 54 Recipe)	10	
Large salad with 2 Tbsp dressing	150	
Glass of wine (4 oz)	100	640 Cal
SNACK		
Graham crackers (2 squares)	60	
Coffee or tea	10	70 Cal
		1520 Cal

Day 55 – 1500 Calorie Meal Plan

BREAKFAST	Calories	Totals
Cantaloupe (½ medium)	50	
Oatmeal (½ cup dry) + ½ cup skim milk + about 15 raisins	220	
Coffee	10	280 Cal
SNACK		
Fresh fruit in season (apple, peach, etc)	70	70 Cal
LUNCH		
Two servings (1 cup) of left over Day 51 salad	270	
Italian or French bread (1 slice)	80	
Lettuce & tomato slices	20	
Hot or iced tea	10	380 Cal
SNACK		
Handful unsalted mixed nuts	100	
Coffee or tea	10	110 Cal
DINNER		
Hearty Vegetable Soup (Day 55 Recipe - page 162)	360	
Italian or French bread (1 slice)	80	
Glass of wine (4 oz)	100	540 Cal
SNACK		
Graham crackers (4 squares)	120	
Coffee or tea	10	130 Cal
		1510 Cal

Day 56 – 1500 Calorie Meal Plan

BREAKFAST	Calories	Totals
Tomato juice (½ cup)	20	
Shredded Wheat (1 cup) + ½ cup skim milk + ½ banana	260	
Coffee	10	290 Cal
SNACK		
Fresh fruit in season (pear, plum, etc)	70	70 Cal
LUNCH		
Roast beef (2 oz) sandwich on whole-grain bread	305	
Lettuce & tomato	20	
Hot or iced tea	10	335 Cal
SNACK		
Coffee or tea	10	10 Cal
DINNER		
Frozen chicken dinner (Day 56 Recipe - page 163)	300	
Large salad with 2 Tbsp dressing	150	
Italian or French bread (1 slice)	80	
Glass of wine (4 oz)	100	630 Cal
SNACK		
Kashi TLC Crunchy Granola Bar	180	
Coffee or tea	10	190 Cal
		1525 Cal

Day 57 – 1500 Calorie Meal Plan

BREAKFAST	Calories	Totals
Cantaloupe (½ medium)	50	
Oatena cereal mix (Day 14 Recipe - page 121)	310	
Coffee	10	370 Cal
SNACK		
Fresh fruit in season (apple, peach, etc)	70	70 Cal
LUNCH		
Salad (3 oz canned tuna, 1 tsp Evoo, onions, celery)	175	
Lettuce & tomato wedges	20	
Italian or French bread (1 slice)	80	
Water	0	275 Cal
SNACK		
Coffee or tea	10	10 Cal
DINNER		
Salmon with Mango Salsa (Day 57 Recipe - p 164)	460	
Large salad with 2 Tbsp dressing	150	
Glass of wine (4 oz)	100	710 Cal
SNACK		
Graham crackers (2 squares)	60	
Coffee or tea	10	70 Cal
		1505 Cal

Day 58 – 1500 Calorie Meal Plan

BREAKFAST	Calories	Totals
Tomato juice (½ cup)	20	
Kashi GoLean (1 cup) + ½ cup skim milk + ½ banana	235	
Coffee	10	265 Cal
SNACK		
Fresh fruit in season (apple, peach, etc)	70	70 Cal
LUNCH		
Soup (Appendix C - page 205)	190	
Italian or French bread (1 slice)	80	
Hot or iced tea	10	280 Cal
SNACK		
Handful unsalted mixed nuts	100	100 Cal
DINNER		
Grilled pork chop w orange (Day 58 Recipe p 165)	470	
Wild rice (¼ cup – after cooking)	50	
Asparagus (7 spear cooked & drained)	20	
Glass of wine (4 oz)	100	640 Cal
SNACK		
Blueberry muffin	145	
Coffee or tea	10	155 Cal
		1510 Cal

Day 59 – 1500 Calorie Meal Plan

BREAKFAST	Calories	Totals
Grapefruit (½)	75	
Scrambled egg	80	
Whole-grain toast (2 slices)	130	
Coffee	10	295 Cal
SNACK		
Fresh fruit in season (peach, plum, etc)	70	70 Cal
LUNCH		
Soup (Appendix C - page 205)	140	
Tomato slices + ¼ cup chopped basil + 1 tsp	50	
Italian or French bread (1 slice)	80	
Hot or ice tea	10	280 Cal
SNACK		
Handful unsalted mixed nuts	100	100 Cal
DINNER		
Eat Out – Fish dinner (Day 59 Recipe - page 166)	530	
Glass of wine (4 oz)	100	630 Cal
SNACK		
Graham crackers (4 squares)	120	
Coffee or tea	10	130 Cal
		1505 Cal

Day 60 – 1500 Calorie Meal Plan

BREAKFAST	Calories	Totals
Grapefruit (½)	75	
Cheerios (1 cup) + ½ cup skim milk + about 15 raisins	190	
Coffee	10	275 Cal
SNACK		
Fresh fruit in season (apple, peach, etc)	70	70 Cal
LUNCH		
Subway 6" (Ham, Cheese + veggies)*	260	
Small salad with 1 Tbsp dressing	75	
Water or diet soda	0	335 Cal
SNACK		
Handful unsalted mixed nuts	100	100 Cal
DINNER		
Chicken Stew (Day 60 Recipe - page 167)	360	
Brown rice (½ cup – after cooking)	100	
Small salad with 1 Tbsp dressing	75	
Italian or French bread (1 slice)	80	
Glass of wine (4 oz)	100	715 Cal
SNACK		
Coffee or tea	10	10 Cal
		1495 Cal

Day 61 – 1500 Calorie Meal Plan

BREAKFAST	Calories	Totals
Orange juice (½ cup)	50	
Wheaties (¾ cup) + ½ cup skim milk + ½ banana	190	
Coffee	10	250 Cal
SNACK		
Fresh fruit in season (apple, plum, etc)	70	70 Cal
LUNCH		
Soup (Appendix C - page 205)	190	
Turkey breast (1 oz) on 1 slice rye bread (½ sandwich)	105	
Water	0	295 Cal
SNACK		
Coffee or tea	10	10 Cal
DINNER		
Shrimp over Spaghetti (Day 61 Recipe - page 168)	450	
Small salad with 1 Tbsp dressing	75	
Italian or French bread (1 slice)	80	
Glass of wine (4 oz)	100	705 Cal
SNACK		
Skinny Cow Ice Cream Sandwich	160	160 Cal
		1500 Cal

Day 62 – 1500 Calorie Meal Plan

BREAKFAST	Calories	Totals
Tomato juice (½ cup)	20	
French toasted English Muffin (Day 2 Recipe p 109)	270	
Light syrup (2 Tbsp)	60	
Coffee	10	360 Cal
SNACK		
Fresh fruit in season (apple, pear, etc)	70	70 Cal
LUNCH		
Salad (3 oz canned tuna, 1 tsp Evoo, onions, celery)	175	
Lettuce & tomato wedges	20	
Italian or French bread (1 slice)	80	
Water	0	275 Cal
SNACK		
Handful unsalted mixed nuts	100	100 Cal
DINNER		
Beef Burgundy (Day 62 Recipe - page 169)	350	
Large salad with 2 Tbsp dressing	150	
Glass of wine (4 oz)	100	600 Cal
SNACK		
Graham crackers (3 squares)	90	
Coffee or tea	10	100 Cal
		1505 Cal

Day 63 – 1500 Calorie Meal Plan

BREAKFAST	Calories	Totals
Grapefruit (½)	75	
Scrambled egg	80	
Whole grain toast (1 slice)	70	
Coffee	10	235 Cal
SNACK		
Greek yogurt (6 oz nonfat, any flavor)	90	90 Cal
LUNCH		
Ham (2 oz) with mustard on 2 slices rye bread	290	
Fresh fruit in season (apple, peach, etc)	70	
Diet soda or water	0	290 Cal
SNACK		
Handful unsalted mixed nuts	100	100 Cal
DINNER		
Chicken cutlet (Day 63 Recipe - page 170)	450	
One small baked potato	50	
Large salad with 2 Tbsp dressing*	175	
Glass of wine (4 oz)	100	775 Cal
* Note Day 63 recipe shows some salad on dinner plate.		
SNACK		
Coffee or tea	10	10 Cal
		1500 Cal

Day 64 – 1500 Calorie Meal Plan

BREAKFAST	Calories	Totals
Grapefruit (½)	75	
Cheerios (1 cup) + ½ cup skim milk + ½ banana	210	
Coffee	10	295 Cal
SNACK		
Fresh fruit in season (apple, pear, etc)	70	70 Cal
LUNCH		
Cottage cheese (1 cup low fat)	180	
Large salad with 2 Tbsp dressing	150	
Water	0	330 Cal
SNACK		
Handful unsalted mixed nuts	100	
Coffee or tea	10	110 Cal
DINNER		
Turkey Meat Loaf (Day 64 Recipe - page 171)	240	
Brown rice (½ cup – after cooking)	100	
Green beans - steamed	30	
Italian or French bread (1 slice)	80	
Glass of wine (4 oz)	100	550 Cal
SNACK		
Skinny Cow Ice Cream Sandwich	160	160 Cal
		1515 Cal

Day 65 – 1500 Calorie Meal Plan

BREAKFAST	Calories	Totals
Cantaloupe (½ medium)	50	
Oatena cereal mix (Day 14 Recipe - page 121)	310	
Coffee	10	370 Cal
SNACK		
Fresh fruit in season (peach, plum, etc)	70	70 Cal
LUNCH		
Soup (Appendix C - page 205)	160	
Italian or French bread (1 slice)	80	
Hot or ice tea	10	250 Cal
SNACK		
Coffee or tea	10	10 Cal
DINNER		
Frozen fish dinner (Day 65 Recipe - page 172)	340	
Large salad with 2 Tbsp dressing	150	
Italian or French bread (1 slice)	80	
Glass of wine (4 oz)	100	670 Cal
SNACK		
100 Calorie Pack Cookies*	100	
Coffee or tea	10	110 Cal
* Such as Nabisco Oreos, Chips Ahoy, etc		1480 Cal

Day 66 – 1500 Calorie Meal Plan

BREAKFAST	Calories	Totals
Tomato juice (½ cup)	20	
Shredded Wheat (1 cup) + ½ cup skim milk + ½ banana	265	
Coffee	10	295 Cal
SNACK		
Fresh fruit in season (peach, plum, etc)	70	70 Cal
LUNCH		
Salad – 3 oz canned salmon, 1 tsp Evoo, onions & celery	200	
Lettuce & tomato wedges	20	
Italian or French bread (1 slice)	80	
Hot or ice tea	10	310 Cal
SNACK		
Handful unsalted mixed nuts	100	
Coffee or tea	10	110 Cal
DINNER		
Pita Pizza (Day 66 Recipe - page 173)	430	
Small salad with 1 Tbsp dressing	75	
Glass of wine (4 oz)	100	605 Cal
SNACK		
100 Calorie Pack Cookies	100	
Coffee or tea	10	110 Cal
		1510 Cal

Day 67 – 1500 Calorie Meal Plan

BREAKFAST	Calories	Totals
Cantaloupe (½ medium)	50	
Oatmeal (½ cup dry) + ½ cup skim milk	190	
Coffee	10	250 Cal
SNACK		
Fresh fruit in season (Apple, plum, etc)	70	70 Cal
LUNCH		
Soup (Appendix C - page 205)	140	
Grilled cheese sandwich (2 slices 2% cheese)	240	
Diet soda or water	0	380 Cal
SNACK		
Handful unsalted mixed nuts	100	100 Cal
DINNER		
Eat Out – Chicken dinner (Day 67 Recipe p 174)	530	
Glass of wine (4 oz)	100	630 Cal
SNACK		
Fiber One Chocolate Fudge Brownie	90	90 Cal
		1520 Cal

Day 68 – 1500 Calorie Meal Plan

BREAKFAST	Calories	Totals
Cantaloupe (½ medium)	50	
Wheaties (¾ cup) + ½ cup skim milk + ½ banana	190	
Coffee	10	250 Cal
SNACK		
Fresh fruit in season (peach, plum, etc)	70	70 Cal
LUNCH		
Soup (Appendix C - page 205)	160	
Turkey (1 oz) on 1 slice of rye bread (½ sandwich)	120	
Lettuce	0	
Water	0	280 Cal
SNACK		
Coffee or tea	10	10 Cal
DINNER		
Pork Medallions lime sauce (Day 68 Recipe p 175)	450	
Green beans - steamed	30	
Large salad with 2 Tbsp dressing	150	
Italian or French bread (1 slice)	80	
Glass of wine (4 oz)	100	810 Cal
SNACK		
Fiber One Chocolate Fudge Brownie	90	90 Cal
		1510 Cal

Day 69 – 1500 Calorie Meal Plan

BREAKFAST	Calories	Totals
Orange juice (½ cup)	50	
Soft-boiled egg	80	
Whole grain toast (2 slices)	130	
Coffee	10	270 Cal
SNACK		
Greek Yogurt (6 oz nonfat, any flavor)	90	90 Cal
LUNCH		
Salad (3 oz canned tuna, 1 tsp Evoo, onions, celery)	175	
Lettuce & tomato wedges	20	
Italian or French bread (1 slice)	80	
Coffee or tea	10	285 Cal
SNACK		
Fresh fruit in season – (apple, peach, etc)	70	70 Cal
DINNER		
Healthy Chicken Salad (Day 69 Recipe - page 176)	330	
Small salad with 1 Tbsp dressing	75	
Italian or French bread (1 slice)	80	
Glass of wine (4 oz)	100	585 Cal
SNACK		
Kashi TLC Crunchy Granola Bar	180	
Coffee or tea	10	190 Cal
		1490 Cal

Day 70 – 1500 Calorie Meal Plan

BREAKFAST	Calories	Totals
Orange juice (½ cup)	50	
Wild blueberry pancakes (Day 10 Recipe - page 117)	190	
Light syrup (2 Tbsp)	60	
Coffee	10	310 Cal
SNACK		
Fresh fruit in season (apple, peach, etc)	70	70 Cal
LUNCH		
Peanut butter (2 Tbsp) on 2 slices whole-grain bread	340	
Skim milk (6 oz)	70	410 Cal
SNACK		
Handful unsalted mixed nuts	100	
Coffee or tea	10	110 Cal
DINNER		
Baked Cod (Day 70 Recipe - page 177)	230	
Brown rice (½ cup – after cooking)	100	
Green beans - steamed	25	
Zucchini, tomatoes & onion – steamed	45	
Glass of wine (4 oz)	100	500 Cal
SNACK		
100 Calorie Pack Cookies	100	
Coffee or tea	10	110 Cal
		1510 Cal

Day 71 – 1500 Calorie Meal Plan

BREAKFAST	Calories	Totals
Fresh sliced orange	75	
Cheerios (1 cup) + ½ cup skim milk + about 15 raisins	190	
Coffee	10	275 Cal
SNACK		
Fresh fruit in season (peach, plum, etc)	70	70 Cal
LUNCH		
Cottage cheese (1 cup low fat)	180	
Small salad with 1 Tbsp dressing	75	
Italian or French bread (1 slice)	80	
Hot or iced tea	10	345 Cal
SNACK		
Handful unsalted mixed nuts	100	100 Cal
DINNER		
Chicken Scaloppini (Day 71 Recipe - page 178)	260	
White Rice (½ cup – after cooking)	100	
Snow peas or green beans - steamed	25	
Italian or French bread (1 slice)	80	
Glass of wine (4 oz)	100	565 Cal
SNACK		
Graham crackers (4 squares)	120	
Coffee or tea	10	130 Cal
		1495 Cal

Day 72 – 1500 Calorie Meal Plan

BREAKFAST	Calories	Totals
Grapefruit (½)	75	
Scrambled egg	80	
Whole-grain toast (2 slices)	130	
Coffee	10	295 Cal
SNACK		
Greek Yogurt (6 oz nonfat, any flavor)	90	90 Cal
LUNCH		
Soup (Appendix C - page 205)	160	
Italian or French bread (1 slice)	80	
Hot or iced tea	10	250 Cal
SNACK		
Handful unsalted mixed nuts	100	
Coffee or tea	10	110 Cal
DINNER		
Eat Out – Fish dinner (Day 72 Recipe - page 179)	495	
Glass of wine (4 oz)	100	595 Cal
SNACK		
Skinny Cow Ice Cream Sandwich	160	160 Cal
		1500 Cal

Day 73 – 1500 Calorie Meal Plan

BREAKFAST	Calories	Totals
Orange juice (½ cup)	50	
Shredded Wheat (1 cup)+ ½ cup skim milk + ½ banana	260	
Coffee	10	320 Cal
SNACK		
Fresh fruit in season (peach, apple, etc)	70	70 Cal
LUNCH		
Turkey frank (2 oz) with mustard & relish	150	
Hot-dog bun	130	
Diet soda or water	0	280 Cal
SNACK		
Handful unsalted mixed nuts	100	100 Cal
DINNER		
Pasta Pomodoro (Day 73 Recipe - page 180)	420	
Large salad with 2 Tbsp dressing	150	
Italian or French bread (1 slice)	80	
Glass of wine (4 oz)	100	750 Cal
SNACK		
		1520 Cal

Day 74 – 1500 Calorie Meal Plan

BREAKFAST	Calories	Totals
Cantaloupe (½ medium)	50	
Wheaties (¾ cup) + ½ cup skim milk + ½ banana	190	
Coffee	10	250 Cal
SNACK		
Fresh fruit in season (peach, plum, etc)	70	70 Cal
LUNCH		
Grilled Swiss cheese sandwich (2 oz low-fat cheese)	320	
Hot or iced tea	10	330 Cal
SNACK		
Handful unsalted mixed nuts	100	100 Cal
DINNER		
Frozen chicken dinner (Day 74 Recipe - page 181)	300	
Large salad with 2 Tbsp dressing	150	
Italian or French bread (1 slice)	80	
Glass of wine (4 oz)	100	630 Cal
SNACK		
Graham crackers (4 squares)	120	
Coffee or tea	10	130 Cal
		1510 Cal

Day 75 – 1500 Calorie Meal Plan

BREAKFAST	Calories	Totals
Cantaloupe (½ medium)	50	
Oatena cereal mix (Day 14 Recipe - page 121)	310	
Coffee	10	370 Cal
SNACK		
Fresh fruit in season (peach, plum, etc)	70	70 Cal
LUNCH		
Subway 6" (Roast Beef, Cheese + veggies)	245	
Small salad with 1 Tbsp dressing	75	
Diet soda or water	0	320 Cal
SNACK		
Handful unsalted mixed nuts	100	100 Cal
DINNER		
Mediterranean Chicken (Day 75 Recipe - p. 182)	200	
Spaghetti squash (1 cup steamed & drizzled with 1	90	
Green beans (¼ lb – steamed)	30	
Italian or French bread (1 slice)	80	
Glass of wine (4 oz)	100	500 Cal
SNACK		
Skinny Cow Ice Cream Sandwich	160	160 Cal
		1520 Cal

Day 76 – 1500 Calorie Meal Plan

BREAKFAST	Calories	Totals
Orange juice (½ cup)	50	
Kashi GoLean (1 cup) + ½ cup skim milk	185	
Coffee	10	245 Cal
SNACK		
Fresh fruit in season (apple, peach, etc)	70	70 Cal
LUNCH		
Soup (Appendix C - page 205)	150	
Italian or French bread (1 slice)	80	
Hot or iced tea	10	240 Cal
SNACK		
Nature Valley Crunchy Granola Bar	95	95 Cal
DINNER		
Grilled Sea Scallops (Day 76 Recipe - page 183)	200	
Corn on the cob – one ear	100	
Tomato slices drizzled with Evoo	60	
Large salad with 2 Tbsp dressing	150	
Italian or French bread (1 slice)	80	
Glass of wine (4 oz)	100	690 Cal
SNACK		
Skinny Cow Ice Cream Sandwich	160	160 Cal
		1500 Cal

Day 77 – 1500 Calorie Meal Plan

BREAKFAST	Calories	Totals
Cantaloupe (½ medium)	50	
Fried egg	80	
Toasted raisin bread (2 slices)	150	
Coffee	10	290 Cal
SNACK		
Fresh fruit in season (apple, plum, etc)	70	70 Cal
LUNCH		
Soup (Appendix C - page 205)	190	
Lettuce & tomato sandwich (Tbsp light mayo)	180	
Cucumber slices and carrots and celery sticks	15	
Water	0	385 Cal
SNACK		
Nature Valley Crunchy Granola Bar	95	
Coffee or tea	10	105 Cal
DINNER		
Chicken w Peppers & Rice (Day 77 Recipe - p 184)	290	
Large salad with 2 Tbsp dressing	150	
Italian or French bread (1 slice)	80	
Glass of wine (4 oz)	100	620 Cal
SNACK		
Coffee or tea	10	10 Cal
		1480 Cal

Day 78 – 1500 Calorie Meal Plan

BREAKFAST	Calories	Totals
Grapefruit (½)	75	
Cheerios (1 cup) + ½ cup skim milk + about 15 raisins	190	
Coffee	10	275 Cal
SNACK		
Fresh fruit in season (pear, plum, etc)	70	70 Cal
LUNCH		
Soup (Appendix C - page 205)	170	
Small salad with 1 Tbsp dressing	75	
Italian or French bread (1 slice)	80	
Hot or iced tea	10	335 Cal
SNACK		
Nature Valley Crunchy Granola Bar	95	
Coffee or tea	10	105 Cal
DINNER		
Trout with Lemon Capers (Day 78 Recipe - p 185)	340	
Wild rice (½ cup – after cooking)	100	
Green beans (steamed)	30	
Sautéed cherry tomatoes (See page 132)	60	
Italian or French bread (1 slice)	80	
Glass of wine (4 oz)	100	710 Cal
SNACK		
Coffee or tea	10	10 Cal
		1505 Cal

Day 79 – 1500 Calorie Meal Plan

BREAKFAST	Calories	Totals
Grapefruit (½)	75	
Scrambled egg	80	
Whole-grain toast (2 slices)	130	
Coffee	10	295 Cal
SNACK		
Small bunch of grapes	65	65 Cal
LUNCH		
Subway 6" (Ham, Cheese + veggies)	260	
Small salad with 1 Tbsp dressing	75	
Diet soda or water	0	335 Cal
SNACK		
Handful unsalted mixed nuts	100	100 Cal
DINNER		
Eat Out – Italian food (Day 79 Recipe - page 186)	540	
Glass of wine (4 oz)	100	640 Cal
SNACK		
Fiber One Chocolate Fudge Brownie	90	90 Cal
		1525 Cal

Day 80 – 1500 Calorie Meal Plan

BREAKFAST	Calories	Totals
Tomato juice (½ cup)	20	
Shredded Wheat (1 cup) + ½ cup skim milk + ½ banana	260	
Coffee	10	290 Cal
SNACK		
Fresh fruit in season (peach, plum, etc)	70	70 Cal
LUNCH		
Left over Italian food from Day 79	260	
Small salad with 1 Tbsp dressing	75	
Water	0	335 Cal
SNACK		
Handful unsalted mixed nuts	100	100 Cal
DINNER		
Vegetable Chili (Day 80 Recipe - page 187)	360	
Brown rice (½ cup – after cooking)	100	
Small salad with 1 Tbsp dressing	75	
Italian or French bread (1 slice)	80	
Glass of wine (4 oz)	100	715 Cal
SNACK		
Coffee or tea	10	10 Cal
		1520 Cal

Day 81 – 1500 Calorie Meal Plan

BREAKFAST	Calories	Totals
Cantaloupe (½ medium)	50	
Oatmeal (½ cup dry) + ½ cup skim milk	190	
Coffee	10	250 Cal
SNACK		
Fresh fruit in season (apple, peach, etc)	70	70 Cal
LUNCH		
Turkey breast (2 oz) sandwich	245	
Lettuce, tomato and Tbsp light mayo	35	
Hot or iced tea	10	290 Cal
SNACK		
Kashi TLC Chewy Granola Bar	140	
Coffee or tea	10	150 Cal
DINNER		
Frozen meat dinner (Day 81 Recipe - page 188)	300	
Large salad with 2 Tbsp dressing	150	
Italian or French bread (1 slice)	80	
Glass of wine (4 oz)	100	630 Cal
SNACK		
Graham crackers (3 squares)	90	
Coffee or tea	10	100 Cal
		1490 Cal

Day 82 – 1500 Calorie Meal Plan

BREAKFAST	Calories	Totals
Fresh or frozen strawberries (1 cup)	25	
French toasted English Muffin (Day 2 Recipe p 109)	270	
Light syrup (2 Tbsp)	60	
Coffee	10	365 Cal
SNACK		
Fresh fruit in season (apple, plum, etc)	70	70 Cal
LUNCH		
Soup (Appendix C - page 205)	120	
BLT sandwich (2 slices turkey bacon, 1 Tbsp light mayo)	245	
Hot or iced tea	10	375 Cal
SNACK		
Coffee or tea	10	10 Cal
DINNER		
Chicken Salad (Day 82 Recipe - page 189)	440	
Small salad with 1 Tbsp dressing	75	
Italian or French bread (1 slice)	80	
Glass of wine (4 oz)	100	695 Cal
SNACK		
Coffee or tea	10	10 Cal
		1525 Cal

Day 83 – 1500 Calorie Meal Plan

BREAKFAST	Calories	Totals
Cantaloupe (½ medium)	50	
Wheaties (¾ cup) + ½ cup skim milk + ½ banana	190	
Coffee	10	250 Cal
SNACK		
Fresh fruit in season (apple, peach, etc)	70	70 Cal
LUNCH		
Ham (2 oz) with mustard on 2 slices rye bread	300	
Hot or iced tea	10	310 Cal
SNACK		
Handful unsalted mixed nuts	100	100 Cal
DINNER		
Hearty Lentil Soup (Day 83 Recipe - page 190)	260	
Large salad with 2 Tbsp dressing	150	
Italian or French bread (1 slice)	80	
Glass of wine (4 oz)	100	590 Cal
SNACK		
Kashi TLC Crunchy Granola Bar	180	180 Cal
		1500 Cal

Day 84 – 1500 Calorie Meal Plan

BREAKFAST	Calories	Totals
Fresh orange sliced	75	
Soft-boiled egg	80	
Whole-grain toast (2 slices)	130	
Coffee	10	295 Cal
SNACK		
Greek Yogurt (6 oz nonfat, any flavor)	90	90 Cal
LUNCH		
Salad – 3 oz canned salmon, 1 tsp Evoo, onions & celery	200	
Lettuce & tomato wedges	20	
Italian or French bread (1 slice)	80	
Hot or iced tea	10	310 Cal
SNACK		
Coffee or tea	10	10 Cal
DINNER		
Turkey Burger (Day 84 Recipe - page 191)	360	
Green beans or asparagus - steamed	30	
Large salad with 2 Tbsp dressing	150	
Glass of wine (4 oz)	100	640 Cal
SNACK		
Kashi TLC Crunchy Granola Bar	180	180 Cal
		1525 Cal

Day 85 – 1500 Calorie Meal Plan

BREAKFAST	Calories	Totals
Grapefruit (½)	75	
Cheerios (1 cup) + ½ cup skim milk + ½ banana	210	
Coffee	10	295 Cal
SNACK		
Fresh fruit in season (apple, plum, etc)	70	70 Cal
LUNCH		
Cottage cheese (1 cup low fat)	180	
Small salad with 1 Tbsp dressing	75	
Italian or French bread (1 slice)	80	
Water	0	335 Cal
SNACK		
Handful unsalted mixed nuts	100	100 Cal
DINNER		
Meat Loaf (Day 85 Recipe - page 192)	290	
One-half acorn squash (baked with ½ tsp maple syrup)	90	
Spinach (½ cup steamed & drizzled with 1 tsp Evoo)	70	
Italian or French bread (1 slice)	80	
Glass of wine (4 oz)	100	630 Cal
SNACK		
Fiber One Chocolate Fudge Brownie	90	90 Cal
		1520 Cal

Day 86 – 1500 Calorie Meal Plan

BREAKFAST	Calories	Totals
Cantaloupe (½ medium)	50	
Fried egg	80	
Toasted whole-grain bread (2 slices)	130	
Coffee	10	250 Cal
SNACK		
Greek yogurt (6 oz nonfat, any flavor)	90	90 Cal
LUNCH		
Soup (Appendix C - page 205)	200	
Italian or French bread (1 slice)	80	
Lettuce & tomato slices	20	
Water	0	300 Cal
SNACK		
Handful unsalted mixed nuts	100	100 Cal
DINNER		
Tuna & Bean Salad (Day 86 Recipe - page 193)	355	
Small salad with 1 Tbsp dressing	75	
Italian or French bread (1 slice)	80	
Glass of wine (4 oz)	100	610 Cal
SNACK		
Blueberry muffin	145	
Coffee or tea	10	155 Cal
		1505 Cal

Day 87 – 1500 Calorie Meal Plan

BREAKFAST	Calories	Totals
Tomato juice (½ cup)	20	
Oatena cereal mix (Day 14 Recipe - page 121)	310	
Coffee	10	340 Cal
SNACK		
Fresh fruit in season (peach, plum, etc)	70	70 Cal
LUNCH		
Leftover meat loaf (½ of Day 85 serving)	145	
Italian or French bread (1 slice)	80	
Lettuce & tomato slices	20	
Water	0	245 Cal
SNACK		
Nature Valley Crunchy Granola Bar	95	95 Cal
DINNER		
Pasta Primavera (Day 87 Recipe - page 194)	460	
Small salad with 1 Tbsp dressing	75	
Glass of wine (4 oz)	100	635 Cal
SNACK		
Fiber One Chocolate-Fudge Brownie	90	
Coffee or tea	10	100 Cal
		1485 Cal

Day 88 – 1500 Calorie Meal Plan

BREAKFAST	Calories	Totals
Tomato juice (½ cup)	20	
Shredded Wheat (1 cup) + ½ cup skim milk + ½ banana	260	
Coffee	10	290 Cal
SNACK		
Fresh fruit in season (peach, plum, etc)	70	70 Cal
LUNCH		
Subway 6" (Ham, Cheese + veggies)	260	
Small salad with 1 Tbsp dressing	75	
Diet soda or water	0	335 Cal
SNACK		
Handful unsalted mixed nuts	100	
Coffee or tea	10	110 Cal
DINNER		
Frozen chicken dinner (Day 88 Recipe - page 195)	300	
Small salad with 1 Tbsp dressing	75	
Italian or French bread (1 slice)	80	
Glass of wine (4 oz)	100	555 Cal
SNACK		
Kashi TLC Chewy Granola Bar	140	140 Cal
		1500 Cal

Day 89 – 1500 Calorie Meal Plan

BREAKFAST	Calories	Totals
Orange juice (½ cup)	50	
Wild blueberry pancakes (Day 10 Recipe - p. 117)	190	
Light syrup (2 Tbsp)	60	
Coffee	10	310 Cal
SNACK		
Greek yogurt (6 oz, nonfat, any flavor)	90	90 Cal
LUNCH		
Salad (3 oz canned tuna, 1 tsp Evoo, onions, celery)	175	
Lettuce & tomato wedges	20	
Italian or French bread (1 slice)	80	
Water	0	275 Cal
SNACK		
Fresh fruit in season (apple, pear, etc)	70	70 Cal
DINNER		
Fish stew (Day 89 Recipe - page 196)	300	
Large salad with 2 Tbsp dressing	150	
Italian or French bread (1 slice)	80	
Glass of wine (4 oz)	100	630 Cal
SNACK		
Graham crackers (4 squares)	120	
Coffee or tea	10	130 Cal
		1505 Cal

Day 90 – 1500 Calorie Meal Plan

BREAKFAST	Calories	Totals
Fresh orange sliced	75	
Kashi GoLean (1 cup) + ½ cup skim milk	185	
Coffee	10	270 Cal
SNACK		
Fresh fruit in season (apple, plum, etc)	70	70 Cal
LUNCH		
Soup (Appendix C - page 205)	140	
Italian or French bread (1 slice)	80	
Hot or iced tea	10	230 Cal
SNACK		
Handful unsalted mixed nuts	100	
Coffee or tea	10	110 Cal
DINNER		
Veal w Mushrooms & Tomato (Day 90 Recipe)	520	
Italian or French bread (1 slice)	80	
Glass of wine (4 oz)	100	700 Cal
SNACK		
Graham crackers (4 squares)	120	
Coffee or tea	10	130 Cal
		1510 Cal

Recipes and Diet Tips

Day 1- Recipe

<u>Chicken with Peppers & Onions</u>

4 boneless and skinless chicken breasts (about 5 oz each)
Coat the chicken breasts in a bottled barbeque sauce. Prepare medium-hot
fire on well-oiled grill. Place breasts on grill, turning them every 4
minutes, for 10 to 12 minutes, or until done. (To check if breasts are done,
the meat should be moist and white with no sign of pink when you cut into
the breast.) Salt and pepper to taste.
2 medium red peppers, sliced
1 medium onion, sliced
Place peppers and onions in pan with 2 tablespoons fat-free chicken stock.
Sauté until stock is reduced. Spray pan lightly with non-stick cooking oil
and cook another 2 minutes. Salt and pepper to taste.
<u>Serves 4</u>. About 250 Calories per serving (for chicken only).

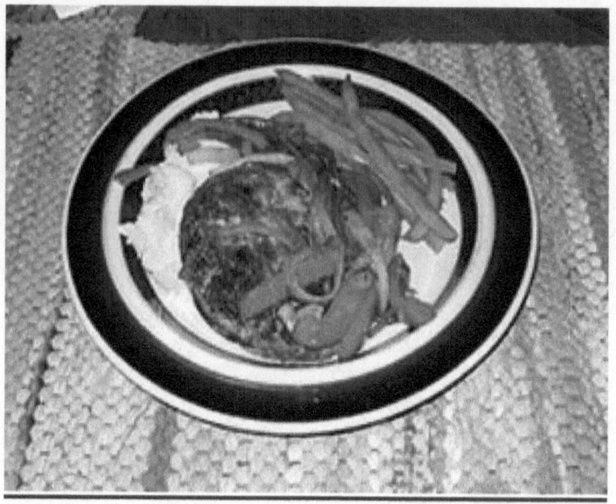

<u>Diet Tip of the Day:</u> Weight Loss – take it one step, one meal, one
workout, one day at a time. Just think of where you'll be in 90 days!

Day 2 Recipe

French-Toasted English Muffin

6 whole wheat English muffins (light)

4 eggs

2 cups skim milk

2 teaspoons (tsp) vanilla

Dash of cinnamon

In a medium bowl, beat together eggs and skim milk. Add vanilla and cinnamon. Separate English muffins into halves and saturate slices in egg mixture. In a non-stick skillet coated with cooking spray, cook muffins until both sides are golden brown. Dust lightly with confectionary sugar. Serve hot or keep in an oven or warmer at 200 °F until ready to plate. **Serves 4**. Three English muffin slices (1½ muffins) per serving. Serving is 270 Calories.

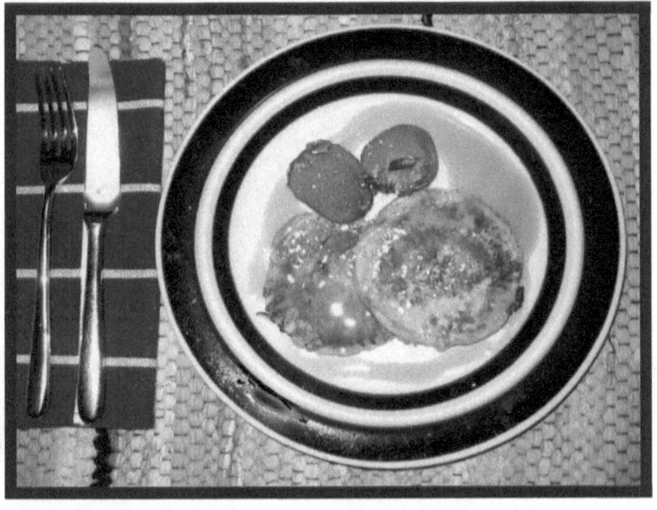

Diet Tip of the Day: "Eat Slowly" This is especially vital when you are trying to lose weight. If you are someone who eats fast, who finishes before everyone else at the table, you are not giving yourself a chance to feel full. While everyone else is still eating, you either sit there and pick, or you have seconds, taking in extra calories you could avoid if you would just slow down.

Day 3 Recipe

<u>Baked Herb-Crusted Cod</u>

4   cod fish fillets (4 to 5 ounces each)
2   tablespoons flour
2   tablespoons cornmeal
2   tablespoons minced fresh herbs
2   teaspoons lemon juice

Sprinkle cod with lemon juice. Mix flour, cornmeal and herbs and dust the cod with the cornmeal-herb mixture. Bake in oven at 375 °F for 10 minutes. Add salt and black pepper to taste.

<u>Serves 4</u>. One serving is about 230 Calories (for cod only).

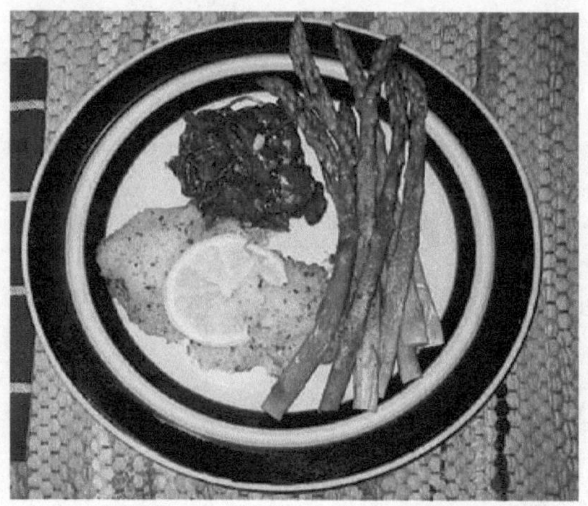

<u>Diet Tip of the Day:</u>. Successful weight loss and subsequent weight maintenance **requires knowledge, desire and discipline**. Avoid the latest fad diets. Instead, take the time to develop a true understanding of weight control and then change your eating and activity habits accordingly.

Day 4 Recipe

<u>Pasta and Veggies</u>

¾ pound penne pasta
2 cups broccoli florets
1 red bell pepper, sliced
1 carrot, cut to 1-inch sticks
½ cup frozen green peas & ½ cup frozen sweet corn
1 small onion, chopped
1 tablespoon minced garlic
3 tablespoons olive oil
1 teaspoon fresh basil, chopped

Cook penne pasta per package directions. Drain and place pasta in a bowl. Pre-cook the carrot and broccoli florets.

In a large heavy skillet, heat the olive oil and sauté onion and garlic until lightly golden. Add vegetables and sauté until the peppers are soft. Combine sautéed vegetables in the bowl with the pasta. Toss well. Garnish with chopped basil, season to taste, and top with freshly grated Parmesan cheese.

<u>Serves 4</u>. 460 Calories per serving

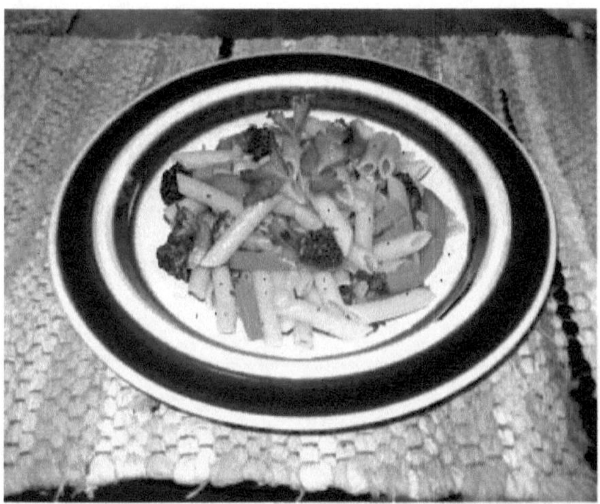

Photo taken before grated cheese was added.

<u>Diet Tip of the Day</u>: When possible, **select fresh and natural foods** and whole-grain products. Avoid chemical preservatives and additives, artificial and imitation foods, refined and processed foods, and foods that are comprised of "nutritionally-empty calories."

Day 5 Recipe

<u>Frozen-Fish Dinner</u>

No recipe today. No cooking today. It's your day off! To find a frozen fish dinner, please go to Appendix A (page 198) which lists approximately 150 frozen dinners manufactured by Healthy Choice, Lean Cuisine and Smart Ones.

Perusing the list, it is obvious that there are not many frozen fish dinners for sale at supermarkets. Note that if you do not use all of the **340 Calories allocated for this Day 5 meal**, use the excess calories anyway you wish. Splurge on extra dessert or save the calories for the next day and have a larger piece of pizza!

Please read the important **Frozen-Food Safety Warning** in Appendix B on page 204.

<u>**Diet Tip of the Day:**</u> **Buy a pedometer** and start walking. For the average person 2,100 steps amounts to walking about one mile. A Harvard study has shown that 8,000 to 10,000 step per day promote weight loss. And you're not obliged to walk continuously until you accrue all 10,000 steps. Rather, all steps throughout the day to wherever and whenever count toward your daily total. Because 10000 steps a day may not be achievable by some people, particularly those who are elderly, sedentary, or who have chronic diseases, rather than insisting on a blanket 10000 steps per day, your initial stepping goal should your baseline steps plus an increment of an additional 2500 steps. (Your baseline being the number of steps you take in an average day.)

Day 6 Recipe

Grandma's Pizza

The following is a pizza recipe used by my Italian grandmother. She was from a small mountain village located between Rome and Naples.

Pizza dough: To save time use prepared dough, preferably whole wheat. Flour a large cutting board. <u>Divide one pound of prepared pizza dough into four parts</u>. Roll out each dough ball as thin as possible.

Tomato sauce: Sauté ½ small onion, chopped fine, in 1 tsp olive oil. Add two finely chopped garlic cloves, 1½ cups chopped plum tomatoes and ½ tsp chopped fresh oregano. Stir and cook about 5 minutes on a low flame.

Pizza preparation & cooking: On each pizza, spread evenly about ¼ cup of the tomato sauce. Add about ½ ounce of shredded part-skim mozzarella cheese, 1 tsp Parmesan cheese, 3 slices of a Portobello mushroom, some torn fresh basil, and drizzle with Evoo. Put pizzas on a pan and place in 475 °F oven for about 15 to 20 minutes, or until crust is crisp and cheese is just melting. (Freeze left over sauce for use on Day 13.)

<u>Serves 4</u>. Make four pizzas. Each pizza contains about 350 Calories.

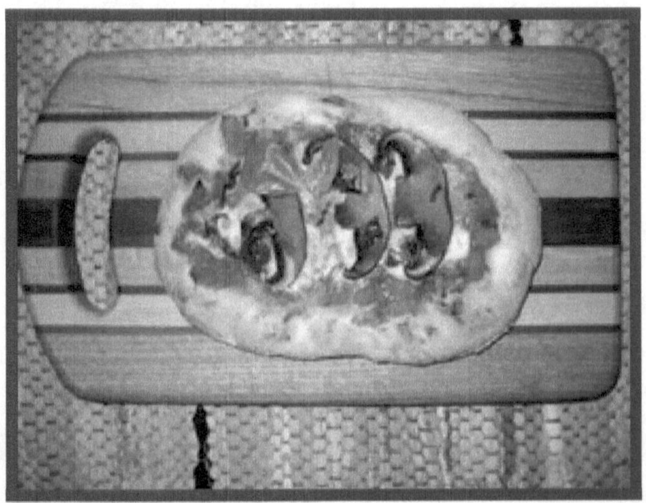

<u>**Diet Tip of the Day:**</u> For **life-long weight control** take a vigorous 30 to 60 minute walk everyday! That's right – everyday. Make exercise a nonflexible top priority part of your life. When it comes to exercise the key words are consistent, persistent, unyielding, dogged. Get the point?

Day 7 Recipe

<u>Chicken Dinner - Out</u>

No recipe today. No cooking today. Have a chicken dinner at your favorite restaurant, but make sure you choose a restaurant where you have a fighting chance to achieve your calorie goal. For 1200 Calorie meal plan, your goal for dinner is a **maximum of 580 Calories**. For 1500 Calorie meal plan, your goal for dinner is a **maximum of 630 Calories**. This includes appetizer, soup, main course, dessert and a glass of wine.

Tips for Eating Out: First, order simple, such as broiled chicken breast with steamed vegetables and brown rice. Tell the waiter you want no sauce, no gravy, nothing added. Then, knowing your calorie objective, and that chicken is about 50 Calories per ounce, most steamed vegetable servings average approximately 50 Calories per cup, and rice is about 100 Calories per ½ cup, decide how much to eat – and take the remainder home. If fresh fruit is not an option, pass on dessert and have the evening snack specified for that day in the diet.

In a restaurant, some nutritionists recommend you eat the low-calorie items on your plate first. Start with the salad, soup and veggies. By the time you get to the chicken and starches you will hopefully be full enough to be content with smaller portions of the higher-calorie choices.

Finally, some dieticians advise their dieting clients not to eat out. That's right. They believe eating at home is safer. But our thought is you have to eat out eventually so why not learn how while your resolve is high?

<u>Diet Tip of the Day:</u> When you're on a diet, eating in a restaurant can be a challenge, because most restaurant portions are huge, and can easily total more than 1,000 Calories. When eating in a restaurant decide how much to eat – and take the remainder home. A good general rule of thumb is to **eat half and bring the rest home**.

Day 8 Recipe

<u>Baked Salmon with Salsa</u>

This is a simple, straight-forward recipe. Again, the advantage of a simple recipe is there are no hidden calories.

   4 5 oz salmon fillets
   6 Tbsp bottled tomato-pepper salsa

Brown salmon fillets in non-stick pan and place in baking dish. Put fillets in an oven preheated to 350 ºF for about 10 minutes. Plate the salmon.
Stir prepared tomato-pepper salsa and spoon it over the salmon.
<u>**Serves 4**</u>. One salmon fillet is about 215 Calories.

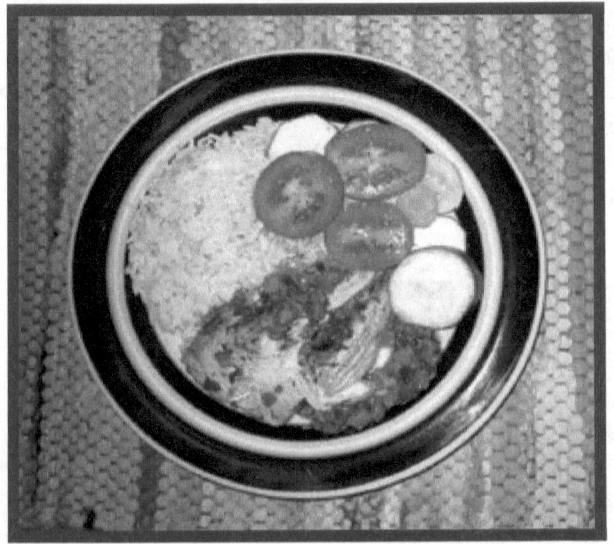

<u>**Diet Tip of the Day:**</u> **Have soup more often.** Most <u>non-cream-based</u> soups are filling and low-calorie.

Day 9 Recipe

Veggie Burger

Vegetable-based burgers can be purchased at your local supermarket. The patty of a veggie burger can be made from vegetables, soy, nuts, mushrooms, textured vegetable protein, dairy, or a combination of these foods.

Two popular veggie burgers are the Boca Burger and Gardenburger. The Boca Burger is made chiefly from soy protein and wheat gluten. (Boca Burger patties are 2.5 oz each and range from 60 to 90 Calories.) The original Gardenburger is made from mushrooms, onions, brown rice, rolled oats, cheese, and spices. (Gardenburger patties are 2.5 oz each and about 100 Calories.)

To prepare, follow package directions. The version shown below has an added slice of low-fat cheddar cheese. The lettuce, tomato and ketchup shown actually add very few extra calories.

The veggie burger patty plus low-fat cheese amounts to approximately 150 Calories. Add a seeded roll and the total rises to 290 Calories.

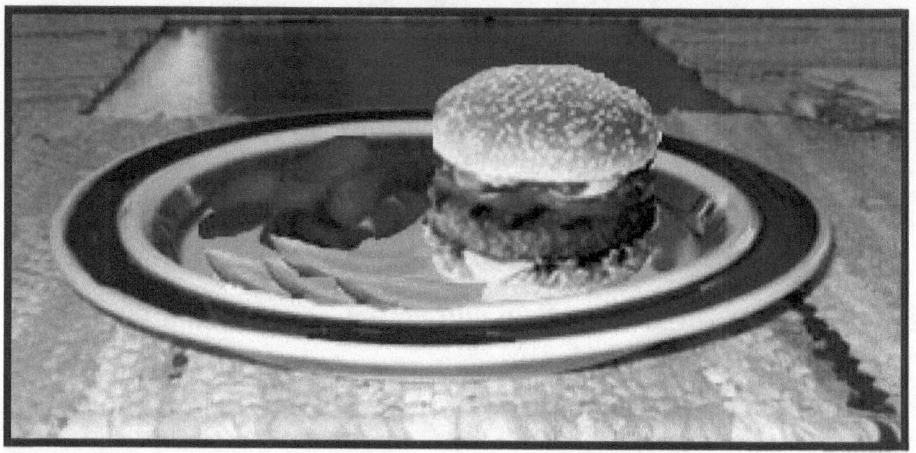

Diet Tip of the Day: **Drink lots of water** – about 8 glasses per day. Add a slice of lemon to make it more interesting. Often, when you think you're hungry, you are just thirsty. So, next time you head for a snack, drink some water first and see if that does it for you.

Day 10 Recipe
<u>Wild Blueberry Pancakes</u>
This recipe makes a relatively low calorie, wholesome batch of delicious
wild blueberry-whole wheat-buttermilk pancakes.
   1 cup whole-wheat flour
   1 cup buttermilk
   1 egg
   1 Tbsp vegetable oil
   1 tsp baking powder
   ½ tsp baking soda
Stir ingredients until blended. Add ¾ cup blueberries and gently stir.
Using medium heat, preheat a non-stick skillet coated with cooking spray.
Pour slightly less than ¼ cup of batter onto skillet per pancake. Cook
slowly until bubbles break on surface of pancake. Turn and cook until
other side is lightly browned. Makes 8 pancakes.
Pictured below are wild-blueberry pancakes with two slices of turkey
bacon.
Serves 4. Each pancake is about 95 Calories

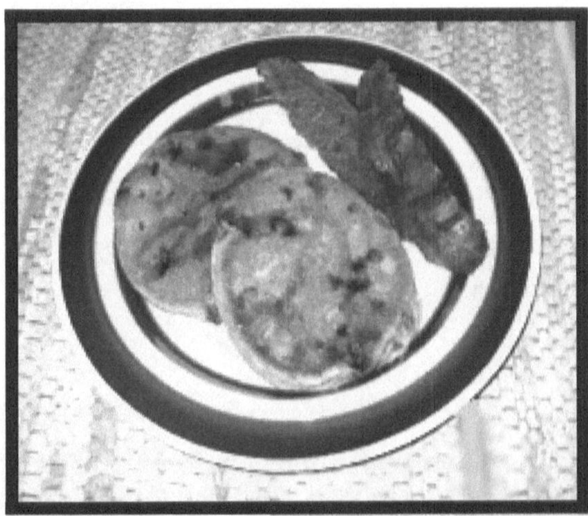

<u>**Diet Tip of the Day:**</u> A peanut butter sandwich on whole wheat bread
with a glass of skim milk and an apple makes a nutritious, reasonably low-
calorie lunch.

Day 11 Recipe

<u>Artichoke-Bean Salad</u>

1 can (19 oz) white kidney beans
10 artichoke hearts, quartered
⅓ cup chopped oregano
⅓ cup chopped parsley
3 cloves garlic, chopped
1 lemon, juiced

Combine ingredients in medium-size bowl. Stir in ¼ cup Evoo. Salt and black pepper to taste.

Serves 6. Artichoke-bean salad has approximately 190 Calories per serving.

Pictured on the plate below are two grilled chicken sausage links with salsa, steamed green beans and the artichoke-bean salad. Incidentally, this artichoke-bean combination over mixed salad greens served with a whole-grain bread makes a delicious, nutritious and reasonable low-calorie main course.

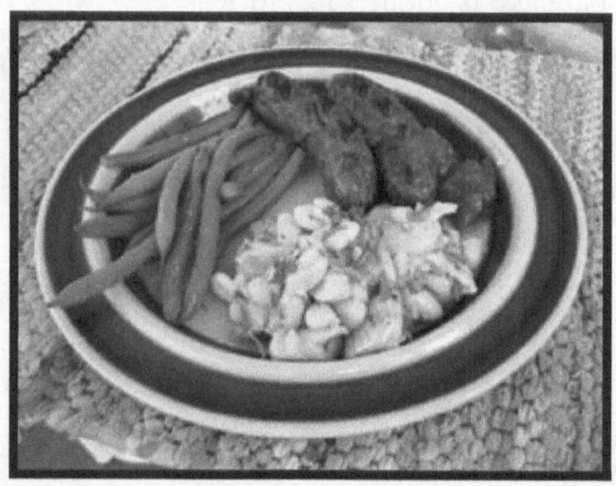

<u>Diet Tip of the Day:</u> Have a small meal before you go to a party. A hardboiled egg, an apple, and a thirst quencher (like water, tea, seltzer, or diet soda) will take the edge off your appetite and make it easier to resist the high-calorie goodies.

Day 12 Recipe

Fish Dinner - Out

No recipe today. No cooking today. Have a fish dinner at your favorite restaurant, but make sure you choose a restaurant where you have a good chance to achieve your calorie goal. For Day 12, your **goal for dinner is a maximum of 595 Calories**. This includes appetizer, soup, main course, dessert and a glass of wine.

Tips for Eating Out: The following is almost an exact repeat of advice given for Day 7. First, order simple, such as broiled fish with steamed vegetables and brown rice. Tell the waiter you want no sauce, no gravy, nothing added. Then, knowing your calorie objective, and that fish is about 50 Calories per ounce, most steamed vegetable servings average approximately 50 Calories per cup, and rice is about 100 Calories per ½ cup, decide how much to eat – and take the remainder home. If fresh fruit is not an option, pass on dessert and have the evening snack specified for that day in the diet.

In a restaurant, I recommend you eat the low-calorie items on your plate first. Start with the salad, soup and veggies. By the time you get to the fish and starches you will hopefully be full enough to be content with smaller portions of the higher-calorie choices.

Diet Tip of the Day: Phytonutrients are found in plant foods such as fruits, vegetables, whole grains, dried beans, nuts and seeds. Unlike protein, fat, vitamins and minerals, phytonutrients are not necessary for life, but evidence is growing that phytonutrients have many beneficial qualities.

Day 13 Recipe

<u>Pasta with Marinara Sauce</u>

Prepare the sauce as you did for the Day 6 pizza. But because the pizza sauce is a bit too thick, add ¼ cup of pasta liquid to thin it. (The spiral pasta shape shown below is called Fusilli, and is a favorite because all the ridges really hold the sauce.)

    ½ pound <u>whole-wheat</u> pasta

    ¼ tsp salt

Prepare the marinara tomato sauce as per Day 6 sauce but dilute it with ¼ cup of pasta liquid. Bring 2 quarts of lightly salted water to a boil. Add pasta and stir occasionally (to keep pasta from sticking to the bottom of the pot). Keep water boiling and cook until pasta are "al dente." (Cooking time is approximately 9 minutes.) Drain pasta, add marinara sauce and serve hot.

<u>Serves 4</u>. One serving is about 225 Calories.

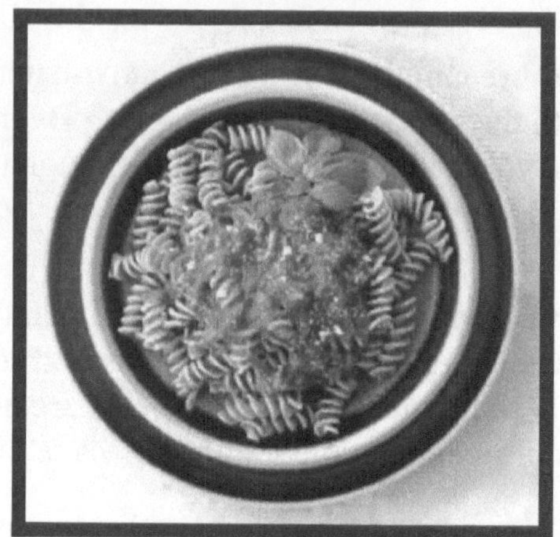

<u>Diet Tip of the Day:</u> **Beware of alcoholic beverages**. Beer has about 13 Calories per ounce, wine 25 Calories per ounce and whiskey 71 Calories per ounce.

Day 14 Recipe
"Oatena" Cereal Mix

Mixing nutritious cereals, hot or cold, is a good way to add variety as well
as nutrition to a meal. This recipe features a mix of two whole grain
cereals: Oatmeal and Wheatena.

    ⅓ cup Oatmeal
    ¼ cup (4 Tbsp) Wheatena
    ¾ cup water
    ½ cup skim milk
    ¼ cup blueberries
    10 raisins

Add Oatmeal, Wheatena, raisins and a dash of salt to a microwave-safe
cereal bowl. Next add water and stir. Place bowl in microwave, on high
power for about 1½ minutes, or until desired consistency is reached. The
result is "Oatena," a mix of oatmeal and Wheatena, shown (half eaten)
below.

Add skim milk and blueberries and serve hot. Because of the natural
sugar in blueberries and raisins, adding sugar is not necessary.

Serves 1. About 310 Calories per serving

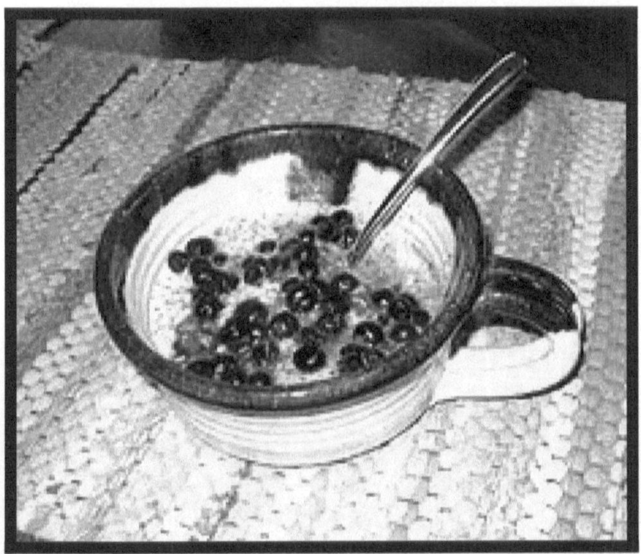

Diet Tip of the Day: Hot or cold cereal topped with fruit, and fat-free
milk makes a nutritious, relatively low-calorie meal anytime.

Day 15 Recipe

<u>Tuna & Bean Salad</u>

1   tuna steak, about 2 inches thick (14 ounces)
2   tablespoons extra-virgin olive oil
1   tablespoon lemon juice
1   garlic clove, crushed
1   tablespoon Dijon mustard
1   15-ounce can cannellini beans, drained
1   small red onion, thinly sliced
2   red peppers, seeded and thinly sliced
½   cucumber, halved lengthwise and thinly sliced
6   cups watercress

Heat a ridged grill pan coated with cooking spray over medium-high heat. Season tuna steak on both sides with coarsely ground black pepper. Cook the tuna 4 minutes on each side - the outside should be browned and the center light pink. Be careful not to overcook. Remove from the pan and set aside.

Mix together the oil, lemon juice, garlic, and mustard in a salad bowl. Season with salt and pepper to taste. Add the cannellini beans, onion, peppers, cucumber and watercress. Toss gently to mix. Cut tuna into ½-inch thick slices. Arrange on top of salad and serve with lemon wedges. **<u>Serves 4</u>**. 355 Calories per serving

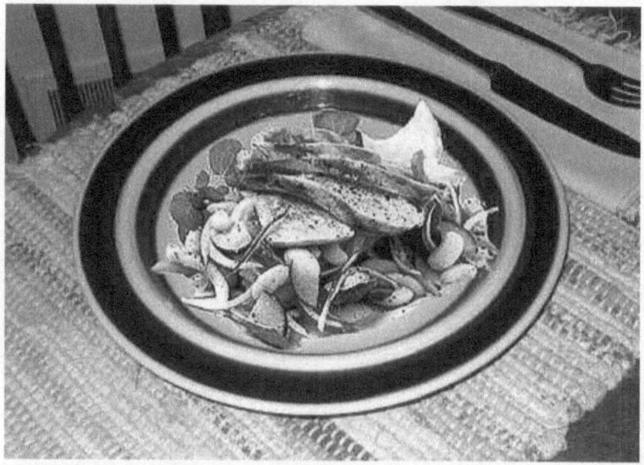

<u>Diet Tip of the Day:</u> In the United States, for a food to be labeled "**whole grain**" it must contain more than 51 percent whole grain by weight.

Day 16 Recipe

<u>Baked Red Snapper</u>

4 red snapper fillets – 4 oz each (salmon may be substituted)
½ cup white wine
½ cup non-fat yogurt mixed with half as much mustard
½ pound green beans
20 cherry tomatoes
4 tsp olive oil
1 cup wild rice, brown rice and wheat berry mix

Prepare rice mix per package directions.

Brown fillets in non-stick pan. Place fillets skin side down in baking dish coated with non-stick spray. Add white wine and cook in oven preheated to 350 °F for about 15 minutes. Spoon pan juices over fillets. Salt and pepper to taste.

Place green beans in skillet. Add ¼-inch of water and cook over medium heat until water boils off. Add cherry tomatoes and olive oil. Stir well and sauté for a few minutes. Season with fresh rosemary and oregano. Salt and pepper to taste.

Plate red snapper fillet and spoon over yogurt-mustard sauce. Add green beans & tomato mix and the wild rice. Serve hot.

<u>Serves 4</u>. One plate consisting of one snapper fillet (215 Calories) with green beans & tomato mix (75 Calories) and wild rice (160 Calories) totals 450 Calories.

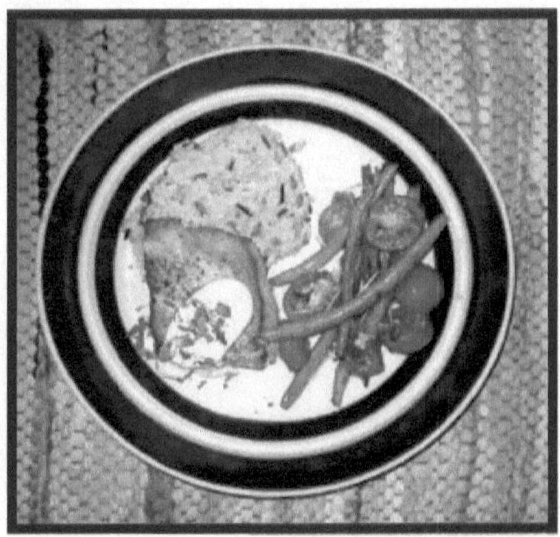

<u>**Diet Tip of the Day:**</u> **Don't have sweets in your house**. This makes them easier to resist. Out of sight, out of mind!

Day 17 Recipe

Cajun Chicken Salad

This is a perfect after-work, quick, nutritious and delicious dinner.

  4 boneless and skinless chicken breasts (about 5 oz each)
  1 bottle Cajun spices
  8 ounces mixed salad greens
  20 cherry tomatoes
  12 pitted black olives

Brush chicken breasts lightly with olive oil. Roll breasts in Cajun spices. Brown breasts on non-stick oven-proof skillet. After breasts are brown, put skillet in 350 ºF oven for approximately 15 minutes, or until done. Cut breasts into ½-inch slices. (When the breasts are done, the meat should be moist and white with no sign of pink.) Serve hot or keep in an oven or warmer at 200 ºF until ready to plate.

Place chicken slices over a bed of mixed salad greens. Add tomatoes, olives and 2 Tbsp of your favorite low-calorie salad dressing.

Serves 4. 330 Calories per serving.

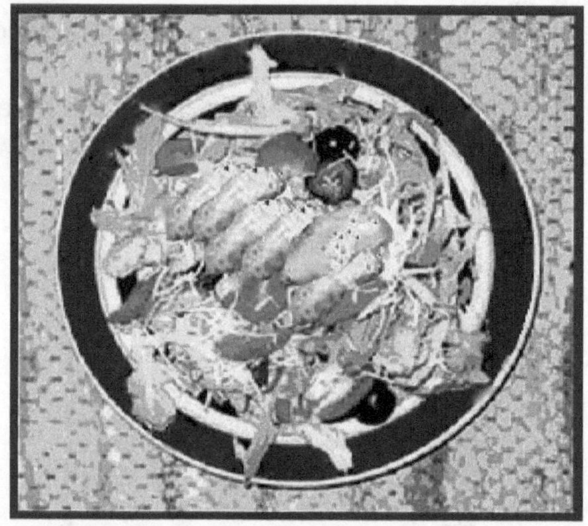

Diet Tip of the Day: Know that **fat-free isn't always your best bet**. Very often sugar is substituted for fat and the calorie total remains the same. Low fat does not necessarily mean low calorie! Rather, look for low-calorie or reduced-calorie products.

Day 18 Recipe

Grilled Swordfish

1¼ pounds swordfish
1 bottle citrus-herb marinade
24 cherry tomatoes
4 medium potatoes
2 cups fresh spinach
1 tsp rosemary & juice of ¼ lemon
2 tsp extra virgin olive oil (Evoo)

Steam spinach with garlic and drizzle with Evoo. Cut up potatoes and place sprinkle with lemon juice, add rosemary, salt and black pepper. Place on grill for about 10 minutes, turning occasionally.

Toss cherry tomatoes in small amount Evoo. Add fresh oregano, salt and black pepper. Place on heavy-duty aluminum foil, seal and grill for about 3 minutes.

Marinade swordfish in citrus-herb vinaigrette. Grill on hot fire for about 5 minutes on one side and 3 minutes on the other, or until done as desired.

Serves 4. One plate consisting of grilled swordfish (250 Calories) with grilled potatoes (100 Calories) and cherry tomatoes (45 Calories) and steamed spinach (50 Calories) totals 445 Calories.

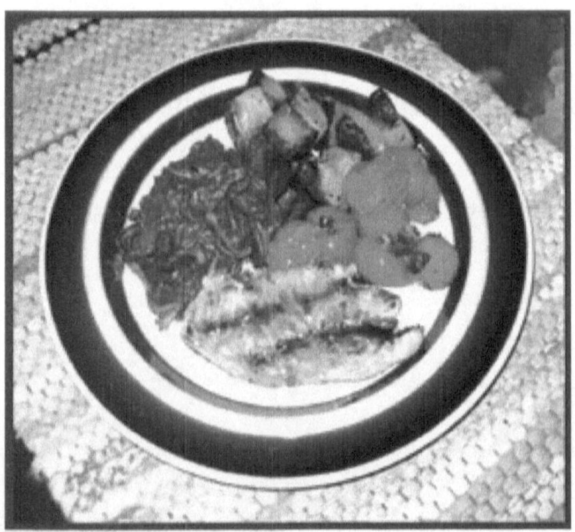

Diet Tip of the Day: Don't be in a hurry to lose weight. Slow weight loss is healthier, is more likely to be permanent, and is easier to sustain over the long haul.

Day 19 Recipe

<u>Italian Food - Out</u>

No recipe today. No cooking today. Have dinner at your favorite Italian restaurant, but make sure you choose a restaurant where you have a reasonable chance to achieve your calorie goal. For today, **your goal for dinner is a maximum of 640 Calories**. This includes any appetizer, soup, main course and a 4 ounce glass of wine.

Tips for Eating Italian: You can consume a lot of calories in an Italian restaurant – if you order carelessly. For example a typical portion is often loaded with about 1000 Calories, then add another 100 Calories for a glass of wine.

First rule, order simple. Look for a dish with lots of vegetables, some fish or chicken. Then, knowing your 640 Calorie objective, and that chicken and fish are about 50 Calories per ounce, most steamed vegetable servings average approximately 50 Calories per cup, and pasta is about 200 Calories per cup, decide how much of the meal you can eat – and take the remainder the diet. Also see Eating Out (page 13) for more guidance.

<u>Diet Tip of the Day:</u>   Another dilemma for dieters is **judging portion size**. It makes no sense to worry about whether to apportion 70 or 80 Calories per ounce for a cut of lean meat if you have no idea whether the portion you are planning to eat weighs four or ten ounces. To be successful, you must learn to estimate portion sizes with reasonable accuracy.

Day 20 Recipe
<u>Quick Pasta alla Puttanesca</u>

This famous pasta dish originated in Naples. Puttanesca means "ladies of the night." The exact origin of the name is unclear, but one thing is clear: It's delicious! Here is one of many recipe versions.

½ pound spaghetti (whole wheat preferred)
20 black pitted olives
1 can (14½ oz) diced tomatoes
½ can (4 oz) tomato sauce
2 Tbsp Evoo
3 cloves of garlic, chopped and 1Tbsp dried minced onion
½ tsp crushed red pepper flakes
1 Tbsp capers drained and rinsed
¼ cup currants

Cook spaghetti according to package directions. Drain and return spaghetti to pot; add a teaspoon Evoo and toss to coat.
Heat 2 tablespoons olive oil in large skillet over medium-high heat. Add red pepper flakes; cook and stir 1 to 2 minutes or until sizzling. Add onion and garlic; cook and stir 1 minute. Finally, add tomatoes with juice, tomato sauce, olives, currants and capers. Cook over medium-high heat, stirring frequently, until sauce is heated through.
<u>Serves 4</u>. About 345 Calories per serving

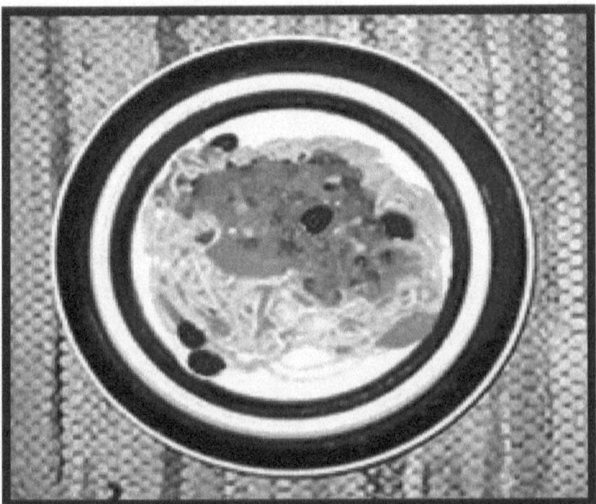

<u>Diet Tip of the Day:</u> Dilute juices, such as apple juice, orange, etc. with water. This cuts the flavor slightly but really reduces calorie content.

Day 21 Recipe

<u>Frozen-Meat Dinner</u>

No recipe today. No cooking today. It's your day off! To find a frozen meat dinner entrée please go to Appendix A (page 198) which lists approximately 150 frozen dinners manufactured by Healthy Choice, Lean Cuisine and Smart Ones.

Note that if you do not use all of the **300 Calories allocated for the Day 21 frozen dinner**, use the excess calories anyway you wish. Splurge on extra dessert or save the calories for another day.

Please read the important **Frozen-Food Safety Warning** in Appendix B on page 204.

<u>**Diet Tip of the Day:**</u> A good understanding of nutrition is not only vital for good health but also will help you control your weight over the long term. For example, did you know that foods that are an "excellent source" of a particular nutrient provide 20% or more of the Recommended Daily Value. Whereas, foods that are a "good source" of a nutrient provide between 10 and 20% of the Recommended Daily Value.

Day 22 Recipe

<u>Shrimp & Spinach Salad</u>

    2 pounds shrimp in shell
    ½ pound small green beans, trimmed
    ½ pound baby spinach leaves
    2 Tbsp lemon juice
    ¼ cup Evoo
    2 tsp minced fresh dill
    1 Tbsp minced green onion

To make vinaigrette, combine lemon juice, olive oil, dill, salt and pepper
to taste and whisk until blended. Stir in minced onion and set aside.
Peel, de-vein and butterfly shrimp. Place shrimp in a bowl and add water
to cover. Add 1 teaspoon of salt, and let stand for 10 minutes. Drain,
rinse, drain again, and dry. Arrange shrimp in broiling pan without a rack.
Brush shrimp with a little vinaigrette and place under preheated broiler,
about 3 inches from heat. Broil about 3 to 4 minutes, turning shrimp once,
or until both sides turn pink.

Remove shrimp from broiler and add remaining vinaigrette and green
beans to the broiling pan. Stir to coat shrimp and beans with vinaigrette.
Pour warm vinaigrette over spinach and toss quickly. Plate the spinach
and arrange shrimp and green beans on top.

<u>Serves 4</u>. 310 Calories per serving.

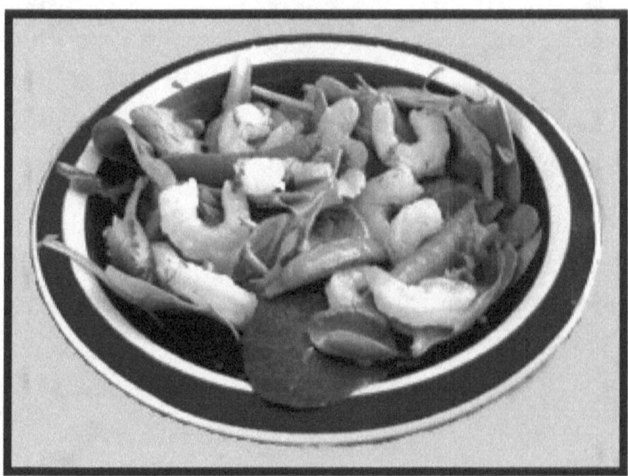

<u>Diet Tip of the Day:</u> After company leaves, have them take some of the
leftover food (particularly the dessert) with them – or take the leftovers to
work the next day.

Day 23 Recipe

<u>Beans & Greens Salad</u>

⅓ cup chopped oregano

⅓ cup chopped parsley

3 cloves garlic, chopped

1 lemon, juiced

Prepare salad dressing by combining above ingredients and stirring in ¼ cup Evoo. Salt and pepper to taste.

½ pound mesclun mix

¼ pound green beans

1 19 oz can garbanzo beans (chickpeas)

Arrange mesclun mix, garbanzo beans and green beans on a large platter. Drizzle salad dressing over beans and greens.

<u>Serves 4</u>. Approximately 260 Calories per serving.

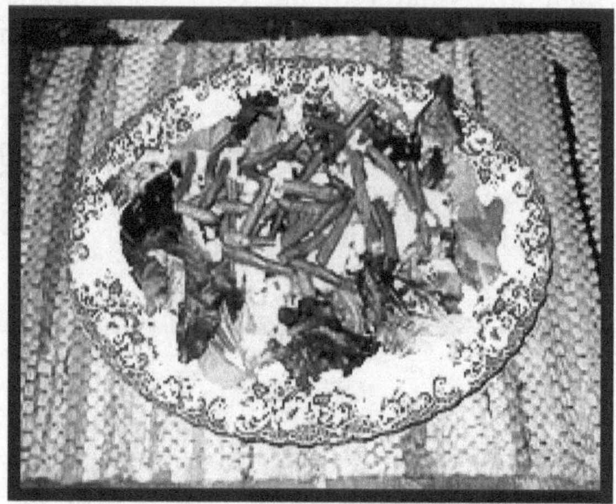

<u>Diet Tip of the Day:</u> Beans are a wonderful food but they are an incomplete protein. If however beans are eaten with a whole-grain bread, the combination forms a complete protein – just as complete and nutritious as meat, poultry, or fish.

Day 24 Recipe

Four-Bean Plus Salad

Note that the total caloric value of the salad will change very little, if the proportions of the bean varieties and corn are varied – according to taste.

  ½ cup canned red kidney beans, drained and rinsed
  ½ cup canned black beans, drained and rinsed
  ½ cup canned chick peas, drained and rinsed
  ½ cup canned cannelloni beans, drained and rinsed
  ½ cup canned corn, drained
  1 small red pepper, chopped
  1 small green pepper, chopped
  2 Tbsp Evoo
  2 Tbsp lemon juice

In a large bowl mix red kidney beans, black beans, chick peas, cannelloni beans, corn and chopped red and green peppers. Stir in Evoo and lemon juice and plate.

Serves about 6. One serving is ½ cup – with about 135 Calories per serving

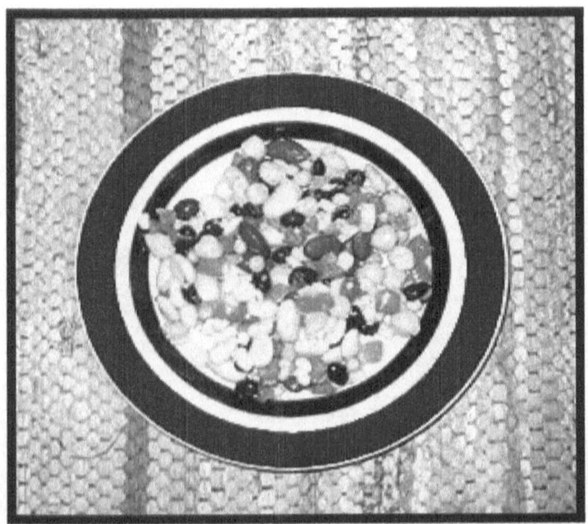

Diet Tip of the Day: Vigorous exercise doesn't necessarily stimulate you to overeat. Just the opposite. In many cases, exercise actually helps curb your appetite – immediately following a workout.

Day 25 Recipe

Pan-Broiled Hanger Steak

1¼ pounds hanger steak, well trimmed of fat
¼ cup lime juice
8 small new potatoes, peeled and halved
12 cherry tomatoes, cut in half
Season both sides of steak with salt and pepper and place in sealable
plastic bag with lime juice. Refrigerate for about one hour.
Boil potatoes about 10 minutes. Rinse in cold water. Sauté potatoes in
small amount of vegetable oil over medium-high heat until brown.
Sauté cherry tomatoes in small amount of olive oil over medium-high heat
until skin begins to crack. Season with chopped fresh basil.
Heat a skillet over medium-high heat. Sear hanger steak on one side for
about 5 minutes. Turn over and sear other side approximately 5 minutes
(for medium done). Pour off any fat that may have accumulated. Carve
into ½-inch slices.
Serves 4. About 320 Calories per serving (for the hanger steak only)

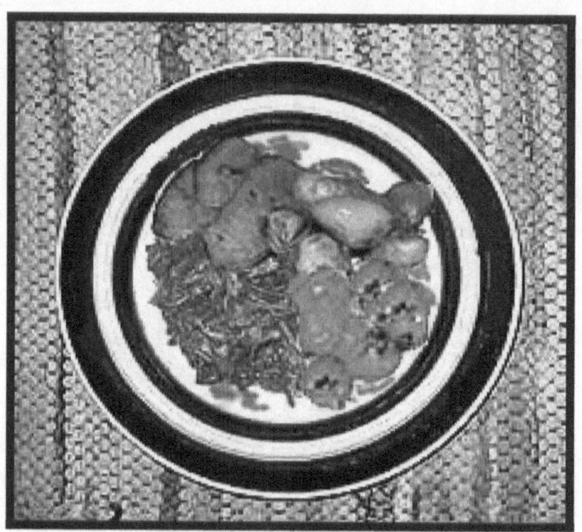

Diet Tip of the Day: If you find yourself at a party, don't stand near the
food! Be aware of the temptation. Make the effort, and you'll find you eat
less.

Day 26 Recipe

<u>Grilled Scallops and Polenta</u>

1 pound sea scallops
¾ cup polenta cornmeal
¾ cup skim milk
1 medium Portobello mushroom
½ pound green beans
¼ cup chopped red onion
16 asparagus spear
1 tsp Evoo

Bring 1½ cups of water and skim milk to rapid boil. Add salt to taste and slowly add polenta while stirring. Reduce heat. Continue stirring until desired consistency is reached. Pour polenta into lightly greased pan. After polenta has cooled cover and refrigerate. Cut chilled polenta into 4 pieces. Grill on medium-hot fire – about two minutes on each side.
Brush Portobello mushroom and asparagus spear with Evoo and place on grill for about 3 minutes on each side.
Grill scallops on medium-hot fire. Turn after two minutes or when first side turns opaque. Grill until second side turns opaque – about another 2 minutes. Don't overcook but test a scallop by cutting to make sure it's cooked through. Salt and pepper to taste.
<u>Serves 4</u>. The food on the plate pictured below totals 380 Calories.

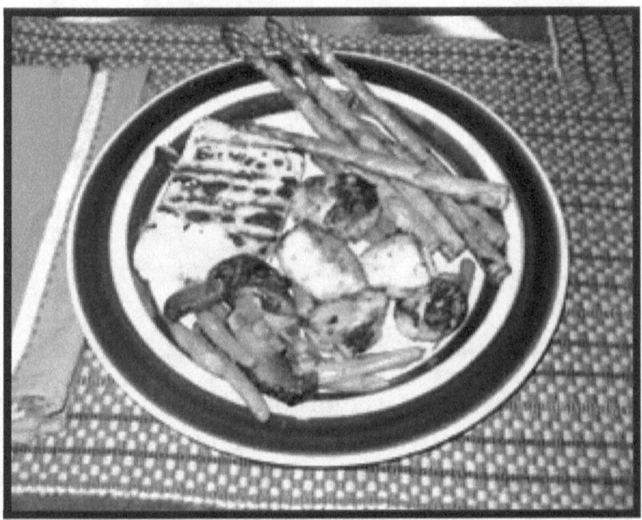

<u>Diet Tip of the Day:</u> To have better control of what you eat **bring your lunch to work**.

Day 27 Recipe
<u>Fettuccine in Summer Sauce</u>

This sauce is often served in the summer because it's lighter than what is usually dished up with pasta. But despite its name the sauce is wonderful year round.

  ½ pound fettuccine

  8 ounces fresh asparagus, trimmed & cut into 2" pieces

  20 cherry tomatoes, halved

  2 Tbsp plus 1 tsp Evoo

  2 cloves of garlic, chopped

  ½ small onion, diced

Cook fettuccine according to package directions. Drain and return pasta to pot; add a teaspoon Evoo and toss to coat. Meanwhile steam asparagus and drain.

In large skillet over medium-high heat, sauté cherry tomatoes in 2 Tbsp olive oil until skin begins to crack. Add onion and cook until translucent. Stir in garlic . Thin sauce with pasta liquid to desired consistency. Toss cooked pasta and asparagus into sauce and serve immediately.

<u>Serves 4</u>. About 290 Calories per serving

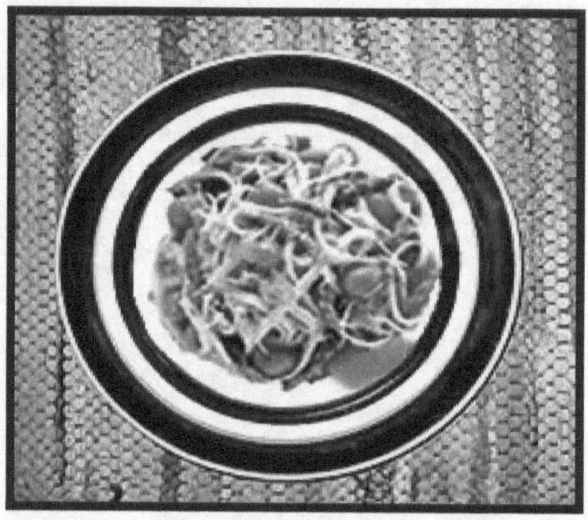

<u>Diet Tip of the Day</u>: A major weight-loss fallacy is that you can get rid of abdominal fat by working your abdominal muscles. This is based on the incorrect belief that fat is eliminated from a particular part of your body if you engage the muscles underneath that layer of fat. No such luck.

Day 28 Recipe

<u>Frozen Chicken Meal</u>

No recipe today. No cooking today. It's your day off! To find a frozen chicken dinner entrée please go to Appendix A (page 198) which lists approximately 150 frozen dinners manufactured by Healthy Choice, Lean Cuisine and Smart Ones.

Note that if you do not use all of the **300 Calories allocated for the Day 28 frozen dinner**, use the excess calories anyway you wish. Splurge on extra dessert or save the calories for another day.

Please read the important **Frozen-Food Safety Warning** in Appendix B on page 204.

<u>Diet Tip of the Day:</u>   The **general weight-change rule is "last on first off."** Assume as you gained weight, the first place you noticed it was on your thighs, next your buttocks, then your face. As you lose weight, it generally will come off in the reverse order, first from your face, then your rear and finally your thighs. And there is not much you can do about that. The truth is there is no food, no exercise, no magic belt, and no pill that will cause your body to lose fat in one place rather than another.

Day 29 Recipe

<u>**Barbequed Shrimp**</u>

  1½ pounds large shrimp
  3 Tbsp bottled barbeque sauce
  4 medium ears of corn

Pour barbeque sauce into shallow bowl. Toss shrimp in barbeque sauce to coat. Place shrimp on medium-hot grill. Turn shrimp after about two minutes or when shrimp turn pink. Grill until second side turns pink – approximately another 2 minutes. Don't overcook but test a shrimp by cutting to make sure it is cooked through. Salt and pepper to taste. Serve hot or at room temperature.

<u>**Serves 4**</u>. About 160 Calories per serving (shrimp only).

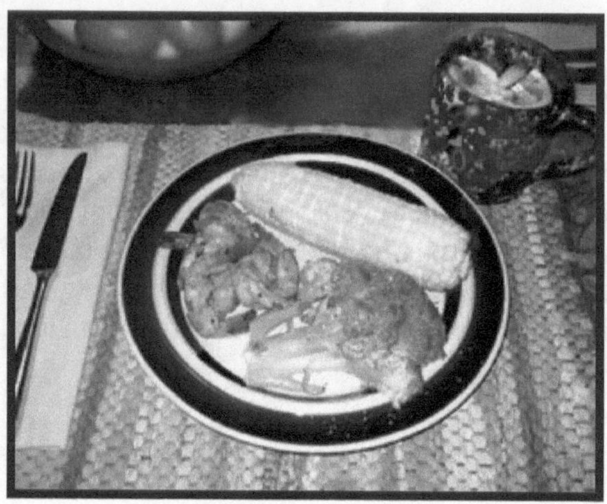

<u>**Diet Tip of the Day:**</u> A very important weight-profile parameter is your waist-to-hip ratio. Health risks for heart attack and stroke increase considerably for men with a ratio above 1.0 and for women with a ratio above 0.8. To calculate your ratio, measure your waist size (at its narrowest circumference) and divide it by your hip size (at the widest wedge).

<u>**Day 30 Recipe**</u>

<u>Pasta e Fagioli</u>

This is one variation of a traditional, nutritious peasant dish served in
Italy.

14.5-oz can whole tomatoes with juice, crushed
14.5-oz can cannellini beans, drained
1 cup of any tube-shaped pasta
2 tablespoon olive oil
1 medium onion, diced
2 cloves garlic, minced
1 stalk celery, finely chopped
3 cups chicken stock
2 cups fresh baby spinach or escarole
1 tsp dried basil
½ teaspoon dried oregano
2 Tbsp fresh parsley, chopped

Heat olive oil, onion and celery in large saucepan over medium heat.
Sauté until onions are golden brown. Add garlic and stir constantly for
one minute. Pour in tomatoes and their juices and bring to a boil. Add
beans and chicken stock and return to a boil. Stir in spinach (or escarole)
and seasonings. Simmer for about 5 minutes. Add pasta and cook about
15 minutes or until pasta is tender but firm. If needed, thin soup with hot
water. Ladle into soup bowls. Garnish with grated Parmesan cheese. Salt
and pepper to taste.
<u>Serves 4</u>. About 300 Calories per serving.

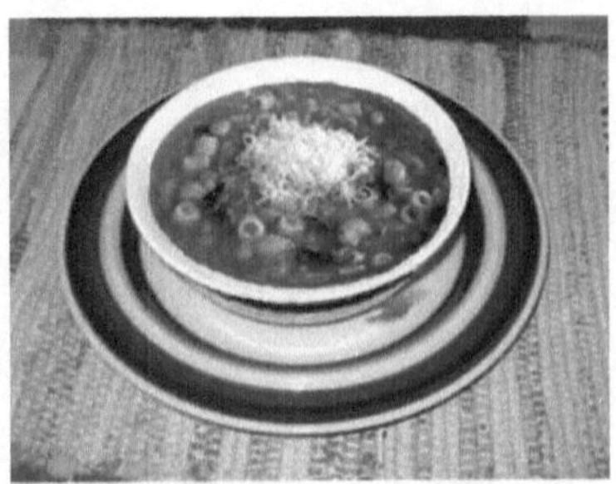

<u>**Diet Tip of the Day**</u>: Pasta alone is an incomplete protein. But when
combined with beans, a complete protein results – that is a protein that
contains all eight essential amino acids.   The dish is every bit as nutritious
as meat, fish or poultry.

137

Day 31 - Recipe

<u>Tina's Baked Sea Bass</u>

   4 4-ounce Chilean sea bass fillets
   ½ pound green beans
   ¾ pint cherry tomatoes (about 20)
   ¾ cup brown rice (prepare per package directions)

<u>Sea Bass:</u> Dust filets with flour. Dip in egg wash & then Panko bread crumbs. Place fillets in baking dish coated with non-stick spray. Bake about 15 minutes in oven preheated to 350 ºF.

<u>Green Beans & Tomato:</u> Place green beans in skillet. Add ¼-inch of water and cook over medium heat until water boils off. Add cherry tomatoes and olive oil. Stir well and sauté for a few minutes. Season with fresh rosemary and oregano.

<u>Brown Rice-Pesto mix:</u> Prepare brown rice per package directions. Add 4 teaspoons packaged "green" pesto. Mix thoroughly.

<u>Red Pepper Sauce:</u> Blend one roasted red pepper (skinned), ½ cup non-fat yogurt, 1 tsp lemon juice, 1 Tbsp olive oil, 1 Tbsp chili sauce, and a dash of Worcestershire sauce.

<u>Serves 4</u>. One plate consisting of one sea bass fillet with spooned over red pepper sauce (150 Calories), green beans & tomato mix (75 Calories), brown rice-pesto mix (120 Calories) and half ear of corn (50 Calories) – totals about 395 Calories.

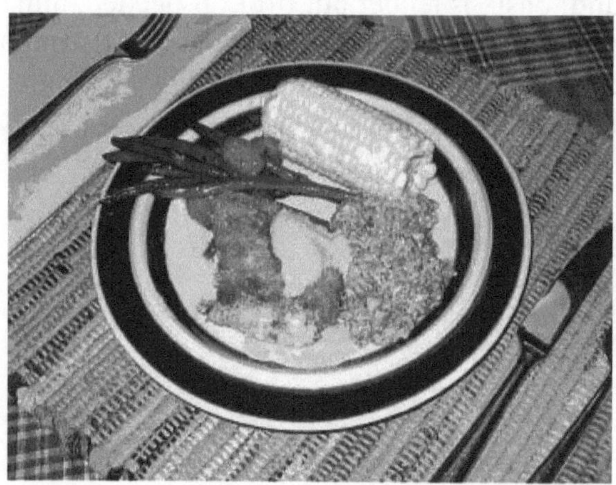

<u>**Diet Tip of the Day:**</u> Protein foods make you **feel full longer** and help prevent overeating.

Day 32 - Recipe

<u>Turkey Tenders & Vegetables</u>

  2   turkey breast tenderloins (about 1½ lb)
  1   medium eggplant (about ¾ lb)
  ¾   pound yellow (summer) squash
  2   medium plum tomatoes, quartered

<u>Marinade</u>: Whisk in a bowl 2 tsp lemon zest, ¼ cup lemon juice, 2 Tbsp olive oil, 1 Tbsp chopped garlic, 1 Tbsp chopped rosemary, ¼ tsp salt and a pinch of black pepper. Put marinade and turkey breasts in large re-sealable plastic bag. Refrigerate about 45 minutes

Slice eggplant and squash lengthwise about ½-inch thick. Place with tomatoes on a baking sheet coated with a nonstick spray.

Grill turkey breasts approximately 7 to 9 minutes per side, or until an instant-read thermometer inserted from the side to middle registers 160°F. Slice turkey and set aside.

Grill eggplant and zucchini about 4 minutes per side, or until just tender. Grill tomatoes about 2 minutes per side, or until charred but not soft. Cut vegetables bite-size and toss with remaining marinade. Serve with sliced turkey.

<u>Serves 4</u>. About 350 Calories per serving (includes turkey and veggies)

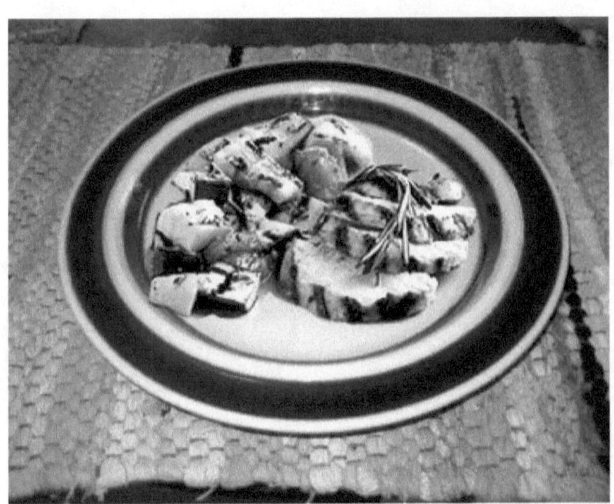

<u>Diet Tip of the Day:</u> It's a lot easier to eat 1,000 Calories than it is to burn 1,000 Calories exercising. So a stroll after dinner isn't going to offset the calories you ingested eating a Big Mac plus fries.

Day 33 - Recipe

<u>Frozen-Fish Dinner</u>

No recipe today. No cooking today. It's your day off! To find a frozen fish dinner, please go to Appendix A (page 198) which lists approximately 150 frozen dinners manufactured by Healthy Choice, Lean Cuisine and Smart Ones.

Perusing the list, it is obvious that there are not many frozen fish dinners for sale at supermarkets. Note that if you do not use all of the **340 Calories allocated for this Day 5 meal**, use the excess calories anyway you wish. Splurge on extra dessert or save the calories for the next day and have a larger piece of pizza!

Please read the important **Frozen-Food Safety Warning** in Appendix B on page 204

<u>**Diet Tip of the Day:**</u> It's amazing how many people tend to confuse thirst with hunger. This often results in overeating when actually drinking water might be the solution. So, the next time you have a seemingly uncontrollable food craving, try drinking a glass of water instead.

Day 34 - Recipe

Pasta Rapini

   2 cloves garlic - coarsely chopped
   1½ cups of crushed San Marzano tomatoes
   2 cups Rapini (broccoli rabe)
   1 tablespoon crushed red pepper flakes (optional)
   ½ pound medium-sized whole wheat pasta

Tomato Sauce: In large pan, sauté two tablespoons olive oil over medium-high heat. Add the garlic and sauté until translucent (but not browned). Add crushed San Marzano tomatoes (use plum tomatoes if San Marzano are not available) and bring to a boil. Reduce heat to low and simmer for about 30 minutes or until cooked. Season with salt and pepper. Set aside.

Rapini: Discard the tough stems and slice into 2-inch pieces. Bring a pot of water to a boil. Add Rapini (a variety of the vegetable broccoli rabe) and 1 tablespoon salt. Blanch Rapini about 5 minutes or until slightly cooked but still crunchy at stems. Drain, set aside and cover.

Cook pasta according to package instructions until al dente. Three minutes before pasta is ready, add the Rapini to the sauté pan (containing the tomato sauce). Heat mixture over medium heat. Drain pasta and add it to the pan with the Rapini and tomatoes. Add hot pepper flakes (optional) and toss for 1 to 2 minutes over high heat. Drizzle lightly with extra virgin olive oil and plate. Delicious!

Serves 4. About 290 Calories per serving

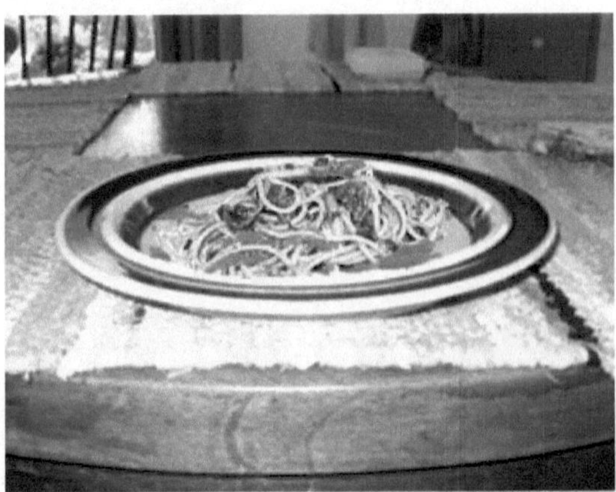

Diet Tip of the Day: Keep a daily food log to **record everything you eat**. For some people it really works wonders.

Day 35 - Recipe

<u>Chicken Dinner - Out</u>

No recipe today. No cooking today. Have a chicken dinner at your favorite restaurant, but make sure you choose a restaurant where you have a fighting chance to achieve your calorie goal. For your chicken dinner out, your maximum allowable calories (includes appetizer, soup, main course and dessert) are as follows:
  - For the **1,200 Calorie Diet**: 530 Calories
  - For the **1,500 Calorie Diet**: 630 Calories

Tips for Eating Chicken Out: First, order simple and order skinless white meat only, such as broiled chicken breast with steamed vegetables and brown rice. (Incidentally, feel free to substitute skinless white meat turkey for chicken.) Tell the waiter you want no sauce, no gravy, nothing added. Then, knowing your calorie objective, and that chicken is about 50 Calories per ounce, most steamed vegetable servings average approximately 50 Calories per cup, and rice is about 100 Calories per ½ cup, decide how much to eat – and take the remainder home. If fresh fruit is not an option, pass on dessert and have the evening snack specified for that day in this diet.

In a restaurant, some nutritionists recommend you eat the low-calorie items on your plate first. Start with the salad, soup and veggies. By the time you get to the chicken and starches you will hopefully be full enough to be content with smaller portions of the higher-calorie choices.

Finally, some dieticians advise their dieting clients not to eat out. That's right. They believe eating at home is safer. But our thought is you have to eat out eventually so why not learn how while your resolve is high?

<u>Diet Tip of the Day:</u> To determine your frame size, circle your wrist with your thumb and third finger. If the tips of your fingers overlap, you have a small frame. If they just touch you are medium, and if they don't touch you have a large frame.

Day 36 - Recipe

<u>Grilled Tilapia</u>

Tilapia is a mild, white fish that inhabits fresh water. This fish has very low levels of mercury because it's fast-growing, short-lived, and mostly eats a vegetarian diet. According to the Monterey Bay Aquarium, choose tilapia farmed in the U.S., in environmentally friendly systems. "Avoid" farmed tilapia from China and Taiwan, where pollution and weak management are a problem.

    4 Tilapia filets (about 6 ounces each)

<u>Marinade</u>: ¾ cup olive oil, ½ lemon, juiced, 1 tablespoons oregano, ½ teaspoon black pepper, ¼ cup red wine vinegar, ½ cup finely chopped parsley, 2 cloves garlic, minced and 2 dashes Tabasco (optional).

Combine all ingredients (except filets) in a large re-sealable plastic bag and shake well. Then place fish filets in the marinade for 30 minutes. Remove fillets from marinade and cook on hot grill for approximately 2 to 3 minutes per side.

<u>Serves 4.</u> About 300 Calories per serving (fish only)

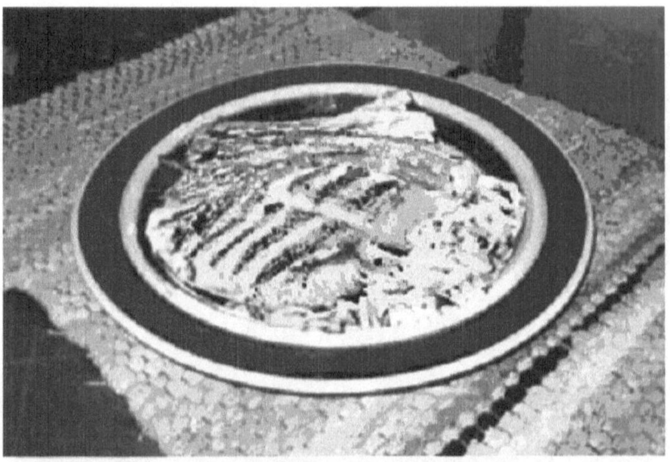

Photo shows two fish filets. Diet serving size is <u>one filet</u>.

<u>Diet Tip of the Day:</u> One serving of asparagus can provide you with 66% of your daily folate needs. Folate is a B-vitamin which is involved with cellular division, and therefore aids the development of a baby's nervous system.

<u>Crab Cakes</u>

    1   lb jumbo crab meat
    1½ Tbsp light mayonnaise
    1½ Tbsp chopped green bell pepper
    2   medium green onions, chopped
    1   large egg, beaten
    1   cup panko bread crumbs
    2   Tbsp canola oil
    ¼   tsp black pepper

Drain crab meat on layers of paper towels. Combine crab meat, bell pepper, mayonnaise, black pepper, onions and egg. Stir in ¼ cup panko bread crumbs. (Place remaining panko in shallow dish.)

Divide crab meat mixture into 8 portions. Shape portions into ¾-inch thick patties and dredge in panko. Place non-stick skillet over medium heat and add 1 Tbsp oil. Add dredged patties and cook 3 minutes on each side or until golden.

Prepare remoulade: Combine ¼ cup light mayonnaise, 2 tsp minced shallots, 1 tsp chopped tarragon, 1 tsp chopped parsley, 1½ tsp Dijon mustard and ¾ tsp wine vinegar. Serve remoulade with crab cakes.
<u>Serves 4</u>. 320 Calories per serving (2 crab cakes)

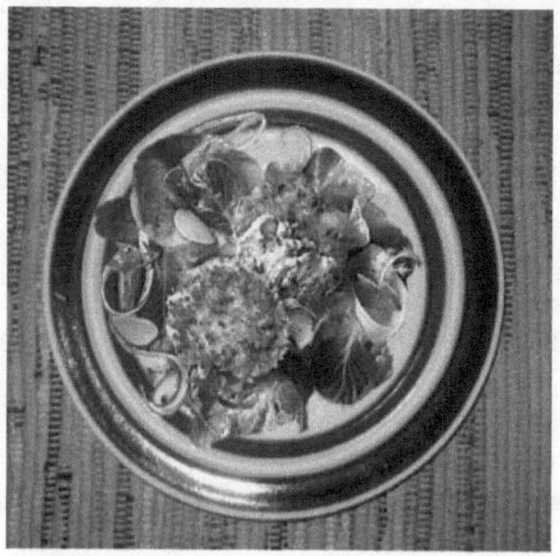

<u>Diet Tip of the Day:</u> **Understanding nutrition** is not only vital for good health but also will help you control your weight over the long term.

Day 38 - Recipe

Pan-Broiled Lamb Chop

Pan broiling is a quick, easy and a relatively low-calorie technique that can be used to cook many meats.

Start with a rib lamb chop about ¾-inch thick that weighs roughly 6 ounces. Next, it is very important to carefully trim all the visible fat. (After removing the fat and accounting for the bone, about 4 ounces of lean meat should remain.)

Season the chop with salt and ground black pepper. Heat a well-seasoned cast iron or nonstick skillet over high heat. Add the chop (or chops) and cook approximately 4 minutes on each side. (Check center of chop with a small incision to determine when the meat is done.)   Plate and serve immediately.

Serves 1: About 320 Calories per chop

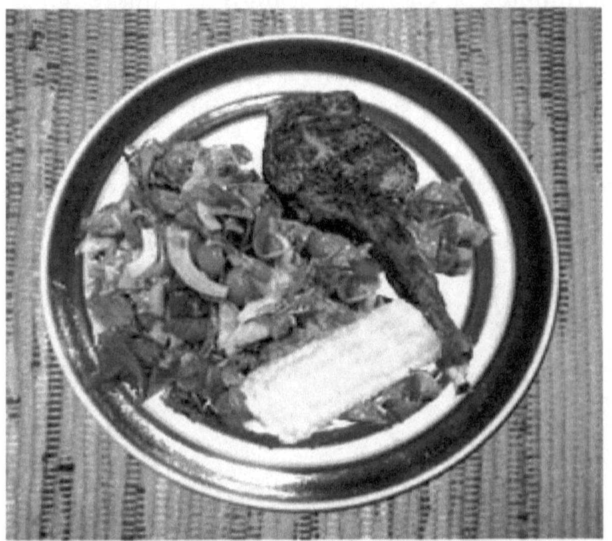

Note corn-on-the-cob is only for the 1,800-Calorie diet.

Diet Tip of the Day: According to a study published in the Journal of Food Chemistry, broccoli, spinach, kale, Brussels sprouts and other dark green vegetables have the highest cancer-fighting potential found in produce.

145

Day 39 - Recipe

<u>Chicken with Veggies</u>

    4 boneless, skinless chicken breast halves (about 5 oz each)
   12 broccoli florets
    1 bunch of asparagus
    2 ripe medium-size tomatoes
    2 tablespoons Lo-Cal (light) salad dressing

Place evenly cut broccoli and asparagus spears in a microwave-safe pan, add a little water to bottom of the pan and top with microwave-safe plastic wrap. (Be sure to pull back one corner of the plastic topper so some steam can escape.) Check veggies periodically and take them out of the microwave when they reach desired softness.

Season chicken breasts evenly with salt and pepper. Heat a large nonstick skillet over medium-high heat. Coat pan with cooking spray. Cook chicken about 4 minutes on each side or until no pink remains.

For each serving, plate one chicken breast and a portion of the steamed broccoli and asparagus. Add one-half of a tomato cut into pieces. Drizzle about 2 tablespoons of a light salad dressing that contains no more than 50 Calories in 2 tablespoons.

<u>Serves 4</u>: One serving of chicken breast halve, veggies & dressing is about 365 Calories.

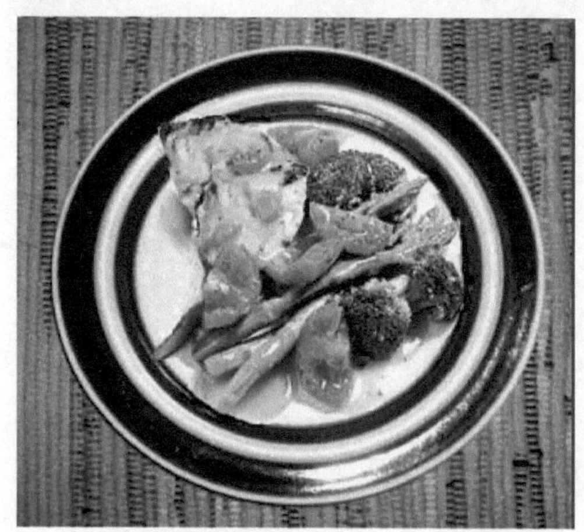

Shown drizzled with Light Thousand Island dressing.

<u>Diet Tip of the Day:</u> Steaming in a microwave oven is one of the best ways to cook veggies so they retain nutrients. Another advantage is the cooking adds no fat or sodium.

Day 40 - Recipe

Fish Dinner - Out

No recipe today. No cooking today. Have a fish dinner at your favorite restaurant, but make sure you choose a restaurant where you have a good chance to achieve your calorie goal. For today, your **goal for dinner is a maximum of 595 Calories**. This includes appetizer, soup, main course and dessert.

Tips for Eating Fish Out: The following is almost an exact repeat of the advice given eating out on previous days. First, order simple, such as broiled fish with steamed vegetables and brown rice. Tell the waiter you want no sauce, no gravy, nothing added. Then, knowing your calorie objective, and that fish is about 50 Calories per ounce, most steamed vegetable servings average approximately 50 Calories per cup, and rice is about 100 Calories per ½ cup, decide how much to eat – and take the remainder home. If fresh fruit is not an option, pass on dessert and have the evening snack specified for that day in the diet.

In a restaurant, some nutritionists recommend you eat the low-calorie items on your plate first. Start with the salad, soup and veggies. By the time you get to the fish and starches you will hopefully be full enough to be content with smaller portions of the higher-calorie choices.

Diet Tip of the Day: For **life-long weight control** take a vigorous 30 to 60 minute walk everyday! That's right – everyday. Make exercise a nonflexible top priority part of your life. When it comes to exercise the key words are consistent, persistent, unyielding, dogged. Get the point?

Day 41 - Recipe

<u>Tina's Healthy Frittata</u>

   3 large eggs, plus 3 egg whites
   ¾ cup reduced-fat cottage cheese
   4 ounces smoked gouda cheese, shredded (about 1 cup)
   1 teaspoon minced fresh rosemary
   3 cloves garlic, thinly sliced
   2 tablespoons Evoo
   1 medium onion, chopped
   16-ounce package frozen mixed vegetables, thawed
   2 tablespoons grated parmesan cheese
   1 scant teaspoon paprika

Position a rack in the upper third of your oven and preheat to 450 degrees F. Whisk eggs and egg whites in a bowl. Add the cottage cheese and whisk until almost smooth. Whisk in the gouda and rosemary. In a 10-inch nonstick skillet over medium-high, cook the garlic in the olive oil. Heat until garlic starts to brown, about 1 to 2 minutes. Add onion, season with salt and cook 2 minutes. Add the vegetables, increase the heat to high and cook until just tender, about 5 minutes. Reduce the heat to medium.

Spread the egg mixture evenly in the pan. Cook, without disturbing until a thin crust forms on the bottom, about 2 minutes. Run a rubber spatula around the edge to release egg from the pan. Continue cooking until the bottom is golden, about 2 to 3 minutes. Sprinkle with the parmesan and paprika. Transfer skillet to the oven and bake about 5 to 7 minutes. Remove from the oven, cover and let sit, 5 to 7 minutes. Cut into 4 wedges.
<u>Serves 4</u>. 320 Calories per serving (¼ of frittata)

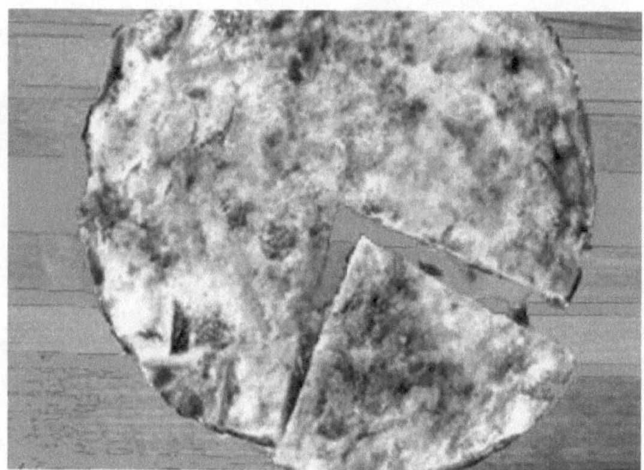

Photo shows frittata on cutting board - hot from skillet.

<u>Dawn's Blueberry Muffins</u>

Wholesome whole-wheat blueberry muffins just like grandma used to make.
Serve them at breakfast, or as a nutritious dessert, or a wonderful snack.
(Make a dozen. Have one today and store the remainder in your freezer until
they are called for again later in the diet.)

    4 ounces bran flakes
    ¼ cup sugar
    1¼ cups whole wheat flour
    1 teaspoon baking soda
    ¼ teaspoon baking powder
    ¼ teaspoon salt
    ½ cup blueberries (fresh or frozen)
    1 egg, beaten
    1 cup buttermilk
    ¼ cup vegetable oil

Preheat oven to 400 ºF. Coat muffin tins with nonstick cooking spray. In a
bowl combine dry ingredients. In another bowl combine wet ingredients and
mix thoroughly. Add wet ingredients to dry ingredients and mix until just
blended. Do not over mix. Gently fold in blueberries. Spoon batter into
muffin tins until two-thirds full. Bake 15 minutes or until muffin tops are
golden brown.

<u>Yield</u> is 12 Muffins, 145 Calories each

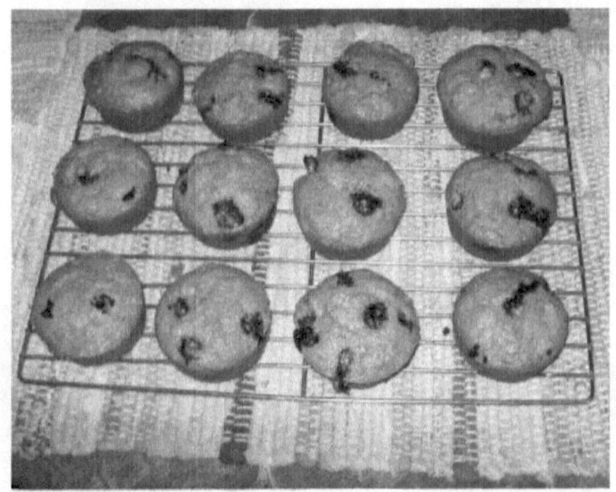

<u>Diet Tip of the Day:</u> **Acquire a good low-calorie cookbook**. Be sure the
recipes cover breakfast, lunch and dinner, and all the recipes contain
nutritional information, especially the calories per serving.

Day 43 - Recipe

Beef Kebob

 1 lb boneless beef tenderloin steaks, 1" thick
 8 ounces medium mushrooms
 2 medium bell peppers (any color), cut in pieces
Marinate ingredients:
 2 tablespoons olive oil
 1 tablespoon chopped fresh oregano
 2 cloves garlic, minced
 ½ teaspoon ground black pepper

Cut beef steak into 1-inch square pieces. Combine marinate ingredients in large bowl. Add beef, mushrooms and bell pepper pieces. Toss to coat. Cover bowl and refrigerate for about two hours. Thread beef and vegetable pieces onto eight 12-inch metal skewers.

Grill kebobs over medium-high heat for 8 to 10 minutes, turning occasionally. Check center of meat with a small incision to determine when the meat is done.

Microwave a one-pound package of frozen mixed vegetables. Plate two kebob skewers and about one-quarter of the mixed veggies.
Serves 4. One plate consisting of two kebob skewers (350 Calories) plus ¼ pound of mixed green vegetables (40 Calories) totals about 390 Calories.

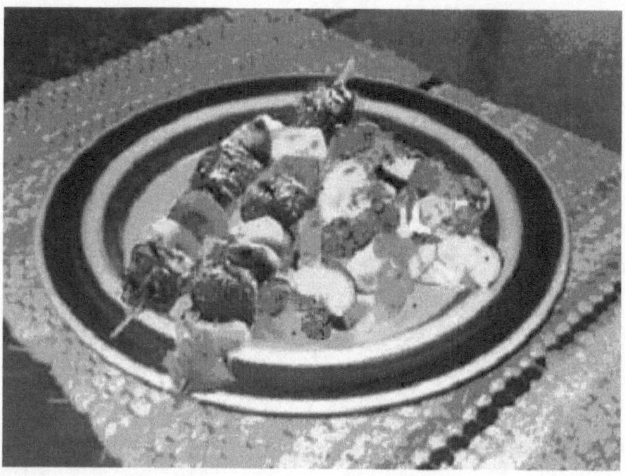

Diet Tip of the Day: Remember your stomach is about the size of your fist. So it doesn't take much food to fill it comfortably.

<h1 style="text-align:center">Day 44 - Recipe</h1>

<u>Baked Haddock</u>

    4   4-oz haddock fillets (or salmon fillets)
    ½   cup white wine
    ½   cup non-fat yogurt mixed with ¼ cup pureed roasted red pepper
    ½   pound green beans
    ¾   pint cherry tomatoes (about 20)
    1   tablespoon olive oil
    ¾   cup bulgur, prepared per package directions

Lightly dust fillets with flour. Dip in beaten egg white and then in Panko bread crumbs. Brown fillets in non-stick pan. Place fillets skin side down in baking dish coated with non-stick spray. Add white wine and cook in oven preheated to 350 ºF for about 15 minutes. Spoon pan juices over fillets. Salt and pepper to taste.

Place green beans in skillet. Add ¼-inch of water and cook over medium heat until water boils off. Add cherry tomatoes and olive oil. Stir well and sauté for a few minutes. Season with fresh rosemary and oregano. Salt and pepper to taste.

Plate haddock fillet and spoon over yogurt-red pepper sauce. Garnish with fresh parsley. Add green beans & tomato mix and the bulgur.   Serve hot.

<u>Serves 4</u>. One plate consisting of one haddock fillet (215 Calories) with green beans & tomato mix (65 Calories) and bulgur (140 Calories) totals 420 Calories.

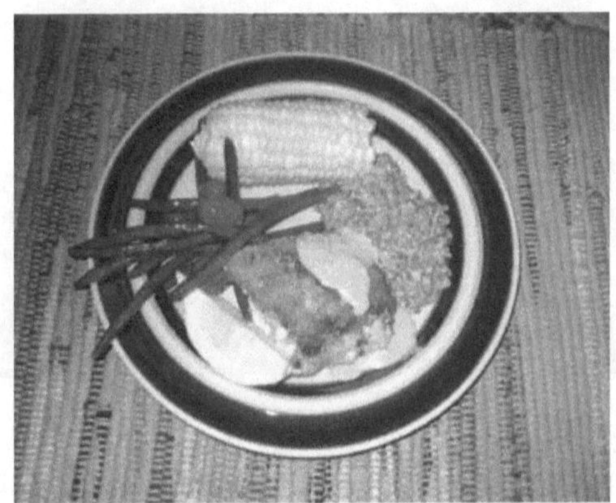

Note that corn-on-the-cob is only for the 1,800 Calorie diet.

<u>Diet Tip of the Day:</u> It's much easier to stay with an exercise program when it's done in tandem. So enlist a friend to be your exercise buddy.

Day 45 - Recipe

<u>Chicken Cacciatore</u>

   ¾ lb skinless, boneless chicken breast halves
   ¼ lb of your favorite pasta
   ½ cup chopped onion
   ½ cup chopped green bell pepper
   14.5-ounce can chopped tomatoes, drained
   8-ounce can tomato sauce
   1½ teaspoons Italian seasoning
   ⅓ cup sliced ripe olives
   ⅛ teaspoon black pepper

Cut chicken breasts into small pieces. Spray a large heavy skillet with olive oil flavored cooking spray.

Sauté chicken, onion and green pepper for 6 to 8 minutes. Stir in drained tomatoes and tomato sauce. Add Italian seasoning, olives and ⅛ teaspoon ground black pepper. Mix well to combine. Lower heat and simmer for 15 to 20 minutes, stirring occasionally.

Cook pasta per package directions. Ladle chicken and sauce over pasta and serve immediately.

<u>Serves 4</u>. About 310 Calories per serving

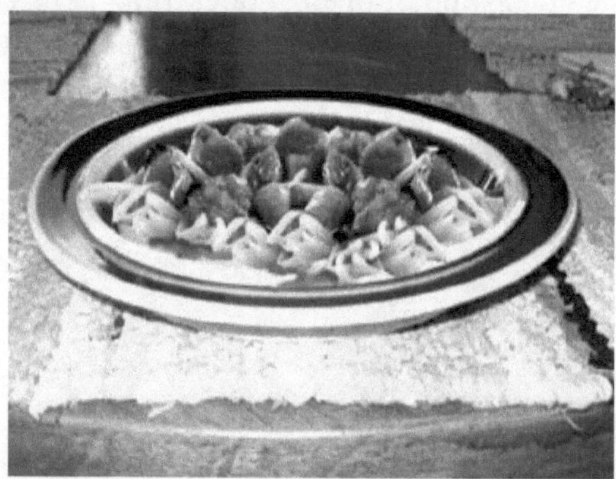

<u>Diet Tip of the Day</u>: Inevitably, you're going to be faced with a stressful situation. Instead of turning to food for comfort, be prepared with some non-food tactics that work for you, such as listening to music, reading, writing in a journal, or meditating.

Day 46 - Recipe

Poached Cod in Tomato Broth

    2   cups dry white wine
    1   cup clam juice
    2   cans (14.5-ounce) diced tomatoes, drained
    1   small onion, diced
    1   garlic clove, minced
    ½   tsp dried parsley, or sprigs of fresh parsley
    1   bay leaf
    12 black olives, pitted and halved
    4   cod fish fillets (about 6 ounces each)

Note that sole, flounder, halibut or haddock may be substituted for cod.

Use a pan large enough to hold the fish in a single layer. Place all the ingredients except the fish in the pan. Over high heat, bring poaching liquid to a boil (pan uncovered). Reduce heat and simmer the liquid another 6 minutes.

Carefully place the fish filets in the liquid. Cover the pan and reduce heat until liquid is just simmering. Poach until fish are completely opaque and tender – about 8 minutes. Plate fish and ladle broth over fish.
Serves 4. 275 Calories per serving.

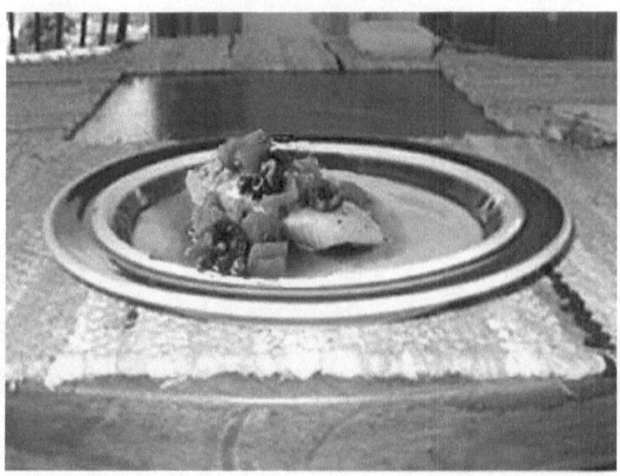

Diet Tip of the Day: **A good reducing diet must help you remain healthy** while you are losing weight.

<h1 style="text-align:center">Day 47 - Recipe</h1>

<u>Black-Eyed Peas over Rice</u>

2 cups fat-free, lower-sodium chicken broth
2 slices smoked bacon
2 cups water
½ teaspoon kosher salt
½ teaspoon freshly ground black pepper
1-pound bag frozen black-eyed peas, thawed
12-ounce bunch fresh turnip greens, trimmed and coarsely chopped
2 tablespoons pepper vinegar

Cook bacon in a Dutch oven over medium heat until crisp. Remove bacon from pan using a slotted spoon, reserving drippings in pan. Crumble bacon.

Add onion to drippings in pan; sauté 4 minutes, stirring occasionally. Stir in broth and the next 5 ingredients (through greens); bring to a boil. Reduce heat, and simmer for about an hour or until peas are tender, stirring occasionally and skimming as necessary. Stir in vinegar. Ladle about 1⅓ cups pea mixture into each of 4 bowls and top evenly with crumbled bacon. <u>Serves 4</u>. 280 Calories per serving (does not include rice)

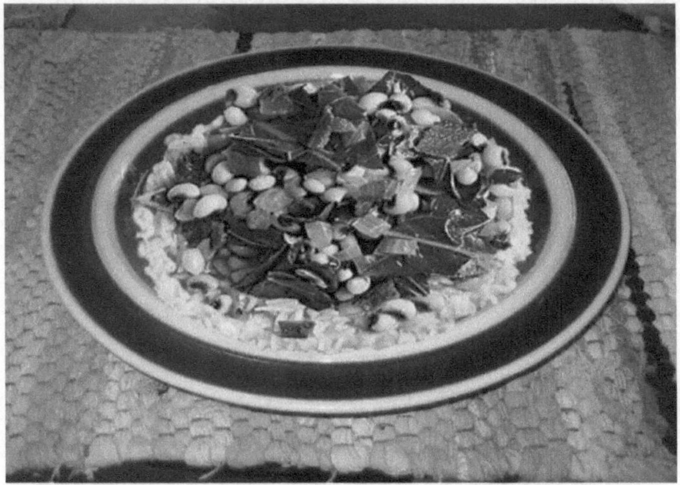

Two servings of black-eyed peas over brown rice on platter.

<u>Diet Tip of the Day:</u> Black-eyed peas are a wonderful food but **black-eyed peas are an incomplete protein**. If however black-eyed peas are eaten with a grain such as rice, the combination forms a complete protein – just as complete a protein as meat, poultry, or fish!

Day 48 - Recipe

<u>Healthy Pasta Salad</u>

½	pound fusilli pasta, cooked until tender but firm
2	broccoli crowns, chopped
¼	pint cherry tomatoes (about 8), halved
½	cup black olives, halved
½	cup garbanzo beans (chick peas)
½	cup fresh "light" mozzarella, chopped
1	tablespoon basil
1	tablespoon rosemary
2	teaspoons garlic powder
¼	cup of a recommended dressing on page 11.

Combine dry ingredients in a medium-size bowl. Stir in salad dressing. Mix thoroughly. Salt and black pepper to taste.

<u>**Serves 4**</u>. 370 Calories per serving.

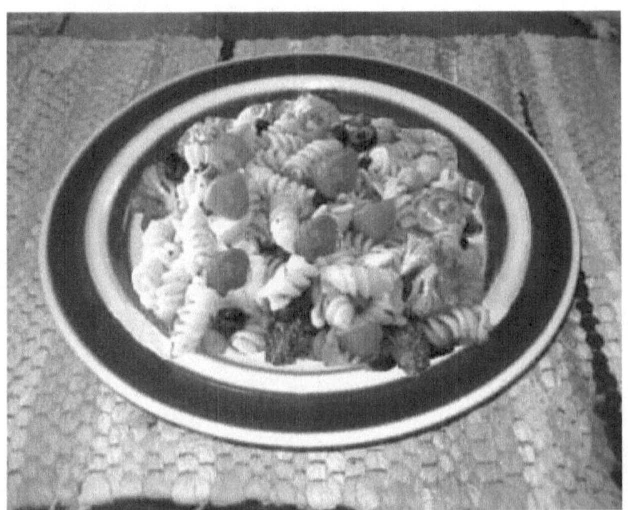

<u>**Diet Tip of the Day:**</u> Ask yourself: "**Why am I overweight**?" Do you eat too much of everything? Too much dessert? Drink too much beer? Is your only exercise walking from the TV to the refrigerator? Determine the why and then focus on one or two of your problem areas. Sometimes it's that simple.

Day 49 - Recipe

Frozen-Meat Dinner

No recipe today. No cooking today. It's your day off! To find a frozen meat dinner entrée please go to Appendix A (page 198) which lists approximately 150 frozen dinners manufactured by Healthy Choice, Lean Cuisine and Smart Ones.

Note that if you do not use all of the **300 Calories allocated for the Day 49 frozen dinner**, use the excess calories anyway you wish. Splurge on extra dessert or save the calories for another day.

Please read the important **Frozen-Food Safety Warning** in Appendix B on page 204.

Diet Tip of the Day: Experts agree that whether you are trying to lose weight or just maintain your weight, **it's calories that count**. It doesn't matter what foods the calories are from. To lose weight you must eat fewer calories than you burn. Calories count! Not carbs, not Weight Watchers points. Calories – period!

Pan-Fried Sole

    4   sole fillets (6-ounces each), skinned
    1   tablespoon olive oil

Salsa Ingredients:
    1 pint cherry tomatoes, quartered
    ¾ cup cucumber, finely chopped
    ⅓ cup yellow bell pepper, finely chopped
    3 tablespoons fresh basil, chopped
    2 tablespoons capers
    1½ tablespoons shallots, finely chopped
    1 tablespoon balsamic vinegar
    2 teaspoons lemon rind, grated

Combine salsa ingredients in a bowl and stir in ½ teaspoon salt and ⅛ teaspoon black pepper. Mix thoroughly.

Heat olive oil in a large nonstick skillet over medium-high heat. Season sole fillets with
½ teaspoon salt and ⅛ teaspoon black pepper. Add fish to pan; cook about 1½ minutes on each side or until fish flakes easily when tested with a fork. Spoon salsa over fish and serve immediately.

Serves 4. 325 Calories per serving

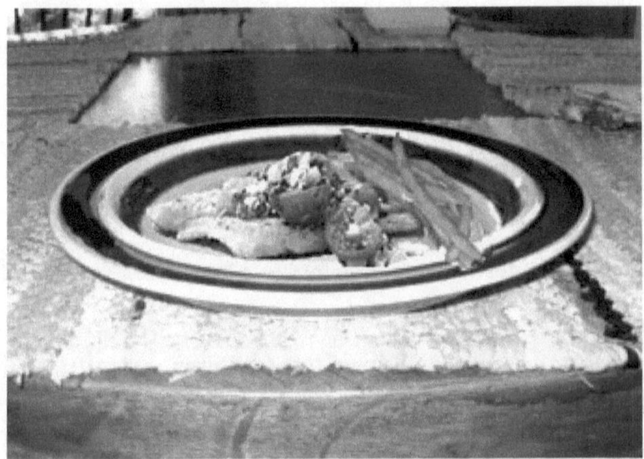

Diet Tip of the Day: If you are overweight start on a weight loss diet now because it will only become **more difficult to lose weight as you get older.**

Day 51 - Recipe

Beans & Greens Salad (Repeated)

>   ⅓ cup chopped oregano
>   ⅓ cup chopped parsley
>   3 cloves garlic, chopped
>   1 lemon, juiced

Prepare dressing by combining above ingredients and stirring in ¼ cup extra-virgin olive oil. Salt and pepper to taste.

>   ½ pound mesclun mix
>   ¼ pound green beans
>   19-ounce can garbanzo beans (chickpeas)

Arrange mesclun mix, garbanzo beans and green beans on a large platter. (Set aside one serving - about ¼ of the salad and ¼ of the dressing for lunch on Day 55. Combine left over dressing and salad when served.) Drizzle the remaining dressing over the rest of the salad.

Serves 4. Approximately 260 Calories per serving.

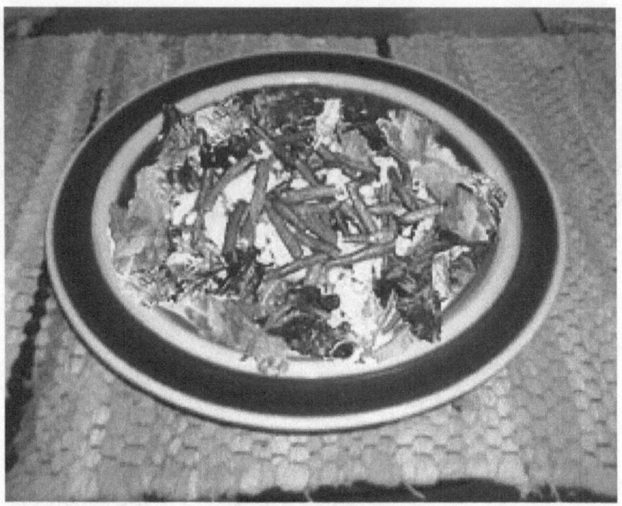

Diet Tip of the Day: Fat-free isn't always your best bet. Low fat doesn't necessarily mean low calorie! Most often sugar is substituted for fat and the calorie total remains the same or even higher. Instead, look for low-calorie or reduced-calorie foods.

<u>Chicken Piccata</u>

- 1 pound boneless skinless chicken breast halves
- 2 teaspoons olive oil
- 1 teaspoon minced garlic
- ¼ cup shallots, diced
- ¾ pound fresh green beans, washed and snipped
- 1 teaspoon lemon juice
- ¼ cup capers, rinsed
- 2 fresh lemons, cut into small wedges

In a skillet, heat olive oil and minced garlic over medium heat. Sauté chicken breasts and shallots for two to three minutes, tossing often, until chicken is partially cooked. Add green beans and one teaspoon of lemon juice and sauté for an additional two to three minutes, or until chicken is completely cooked and green beans are al dente. Add capers; and cover chicken. Let sit for one more minute to warm capers. Serve immediately with wedges of lemon.

<u>Serves 4</u>. 270 calories per serving

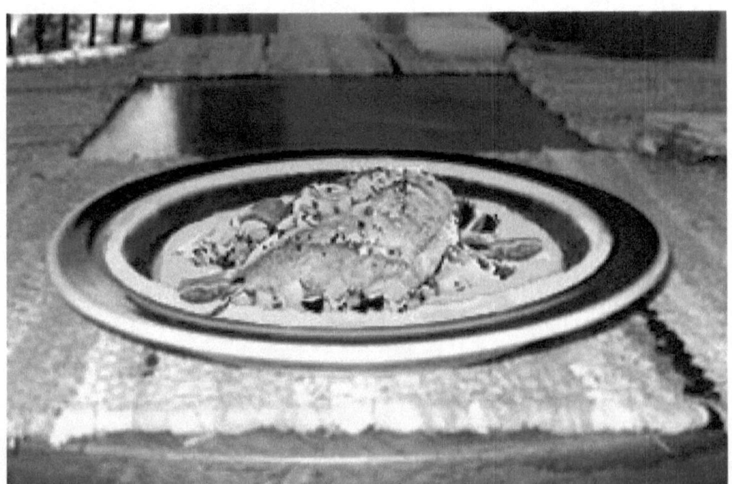

<u>Diet Tip of the Day:</u> Handle **occasional overeating by compensating**. To do this, estimate how far you have strayed from your weight-loss diet and then make amends at the next opportunity (usually the next meal or two) – by eating less.

Day 53 - Recipe

<u>Pasta Primavera</u>

- ½ pound fusilli whole-wheat pasta
- 2 small yellow squash, halved and cut into ½-inch-thick slices
- 1 medium orange bell pepper, cut into 1-inch pieces
- 8 oz. small broccoli florets (3 cups)
- 2 cups halved cherry tomatoes
- 8 green onions, thinly sliced (½ cup)
- 3 Tbs. olive oil
- 3 cloves garlic, minced (about 1 Tbsp)
- ½ cup torn fresh basil leaves
- 1 tsp. grated lemon zest

Combine oil, garlic, and lemon zest in small bowl. Set aside. Cook pasta in large pot of boiling, salted water according to package directions.   Add squash and bell pepper 4 minutes before end of cooking time. Add broccoli 3 minutes before end of cooking time. Drain pasta and vegetables, reserving ½ cup cooking water.

Return pasta mixture to pot, and stir in tomatoes, green onions, basil, oil mixture, and reserved cooking water. Heat over medium-low heat until tomatoes are hot. Serve with Parmesan cheese, if desired.
<u>Serves 4</u>. 350 Calories per serving

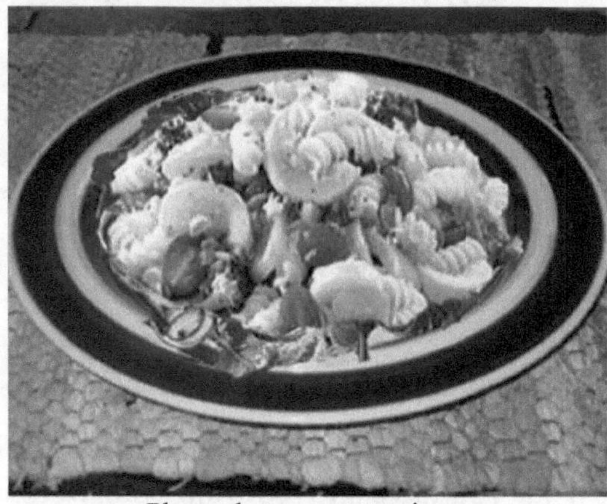
Photo shows two servings.

<u>Diet Tip of the Day:</u> Beware of alcoholic beverages. Beer has about 13 Calories per ounce, wine 25 Calories per ounce and whiskey a whopping 71 Calories per ounce.

Day 54 - Recipe

<u>Tina's Grilled Scallops &Polenta</u>

1 pound sea scallops
¾ cup polenta cornmeal
¾ cup skim milk
1 medium Portobello mushroom
½ pound green beans
¼ cup chopped red onion
16 asparagus spears
1 teaspoon extra-virgin olive oil

Bring 1½ cups of water and skim milk to rapid boil. Add salt to taste and slowly add polenta while stirring. Reduce heat. Continue stirring until desired consistency is reached. Pour polenta into lightly greased pan. After polenta has cooled cover and refrigerate. Cut chilled polenta into 4 pieces. Grill on medium-hot fire – about two minutes on each side.

Brush Portobello mushroom and asparagus spears with olive oil and place on grill for about 3 minutes on each side.

Grill scallops on medium-hot fire. Turn after two minutes or when first side turns opaque. Grill until second side turns opaque – about another 2 minutes. Don't overcook but test a scallop by cutting to make sure it's cooked through. Salt and pepper to taste.

<u>Serves 4</u>. The food on the plate pictured below totals about 380 Calories.

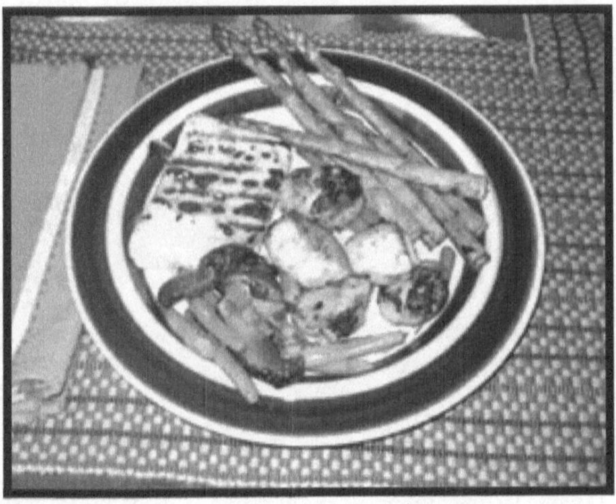

<u>**Diet Tip of the Day:**</u> To have better control of what you eat **bring your lunch to work.**

Day 55 - Recipe

<u>Hearty Vegetable Soup</u>

2 15-oz cans white kidney beans, drained
1 tablespoon olive oil
½ large yellow onion, chopped
2 garlic cloves, minced
1 cup chopped fresh tomatoes
2 celery stalks, cut into ½-inch pieces
1½ carrots, cut into ½-inch pieces
5 cups vegetable stock
1 medium potato, cut into ½-inch pieces
¼ cup chopped fresh basil
¼ head of red cabbage, cut into ½-inch pieces
2 zucchini or summer squash, cut into ½-inch pieces

Heat olive oil in a large pot over medium heat. Add onion and garlic. Sauté 5 minutes. Add green cabbage, tomatoes, celery, and carrots. Sauté 10 minutes. Add beans, 5 cups of stock, potatoes, and basil. Bring to a boil. Reduce heat, cover and simmer for one hour. Add red cabbage, zucchini and salt . Cover and simmer until vegetables are tender, about 20 minutes longer. Stir in about ¼ cup Parmesan cheese and sprinkle a dash of Tabasco hot sauce if you want a little zip

<u>Serves 4</u>. 360 Calories per serving

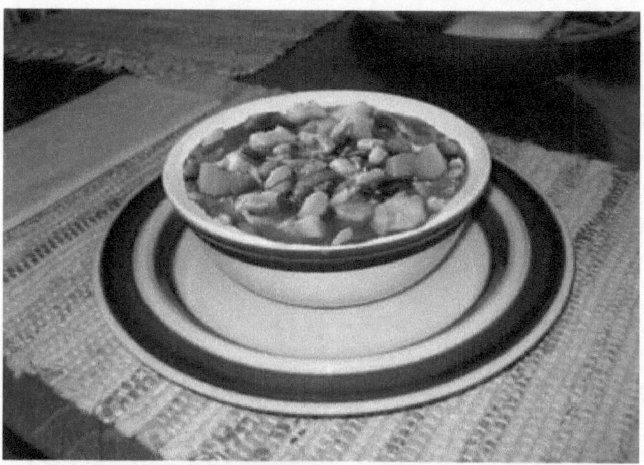

<u>Diet Tip of the Day:</u> Water and fiber contain no calories – that is **zero Calories** per ounce.

Day 56 - Recipe

<u>Frozen Chicken Dinner</u>

No recipe today. No cooking today. It's your day off! To find a frozen chicken dinner entrée please go to Appendix A (page 198) which lists approximately 150 frozen dinners manufactured by Healthy Choice, Lean Cuisine and Smart Ones.

Note that if you do not use all of the **300 Calories allocated for the Day 56 frozen dinner**, use the excess calories anyway you wish. Splurge on extra dessert or save the calories for another day.

Please read the important **Frozen-Food Safety Warning** in Appendix B on page 204.

<u>**Diet Tip of the Day**</u>: To prevent or delay the onset of type II diabetes, experts urge the overweight to lose weight and work out regularly. Weight loss helps your body use insulin more efficiently, and exercise helps metabolize excess circulating blood glucose.

Day 57 - Recipe

<u>Salmon with Mango Salsa</u>

  4 salmon fillets (about 5 ounces each)
  1½ pounds baby new potatoes, halved
  1 mango, ripe
  3 green onions, finely chopped
  3 tablespoons chopped fresh cilantro
  2 tablespoons lemon juice
  2 teaspoons extra-virgin olive oil
  4 cups watercress

Remove any tiny bones from salmon. Press crushed peppercorns into flesh side of salmon. Set aside. Place halved potatoes into saucepan. Cover with water and bring to a boil. Reduce the heat and simmer until tender, about 10-12 minutes and drain.

Prepare salsa: Peel and seed the mango. Dice the mango flesh and put into a large bowl. Mix in green onions, cilantro, lemon juice, olive oil, and an optional dash of Tabasco.

Heat a grill pan coated with nonstick cooking spray over medium-high heat. Place salmon fillets in pan, skin-side down. Cook for 4 minutes. Turn fish over and cook until done, about another 4 minutes. Arrange watercress and new potatoes on serving plates. Place salmon on top and spoon over mango salsa.

<u>Serves 4</u>. 460 Calories per serving

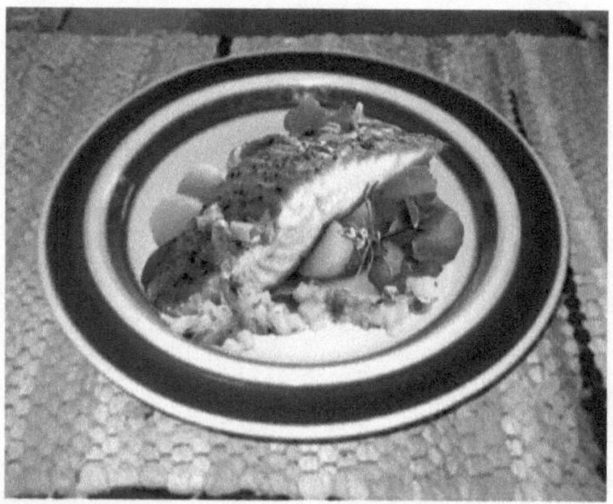

<u>Diet Tip of the Day:</u> All **foods are a combination of water, carbohydrate, protein, fat and fiber**. Knowing this can lead to a better understanding of why a food has a particular caloric value.

<h1 style="text-align:center">Day 58 - Recipe</h1>

<u>Pork Chop with Orange Slices</u>

4 loin pork chops, ½-inch-thick (about 1½ lbs total, including bones)
8 orange slices, ¼-inch-thick
1 teaspoon salt
¾ teaspoon black pepper
¼ cup orange marmalade preserve
½ cup bottled fruit-based barbecue sauce
such as Grandville's Gourmet BBQ Sauce

<u>Marinade</u>: ½ cup orange juice, 2 teaspoons soy sauce and ¼ teaspoon crushed red pepper.

Combine pork chops and marinade in large re-sealable plastic bag. Refrigerate for about 30 minutes. Remove chops from marinade and season with salt and black pepper.

Stir together orange marmalade and BBQ sauce in a small bowl. Brush one side of pork chops evenly with half of marmalade-BBQ mixture. Grill chops, with marmalade-BBQ mixture side up over medium-high heat (about 375°) for about 5 minutes or until done. Turn chops, and brush with remaining marmalade-BBQ mixture. Grill another 5 minutes or until done. Grill orange slices over medium-high heat, 1 minute on each side.
<u>**Serves 4**</u>. 470 Calories per serving (includes pork chop and two orange slices).

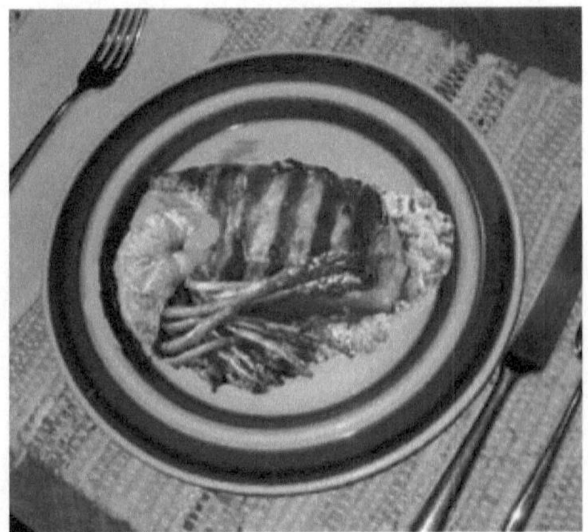

<u>**Diet Tip of the Day:**</u> Make sure fat is trimmed from meat. Most meats are about 80 Calories per ounce – whereas, pure fat is 256 Calories per ounce!

Day 59 - Recipe

<u>Fish Dinner - Out</u>

No recipe today. No cooking today. Have a fish dinner at your favorite restaurant, but make sure you choose a restaurant where you have a good chance to achieve your calorie goal. For today, your **goal for dinner is a maximum of 595 Calories**. This includes appetizer, soup, main course and dessert.

Tips for Eating Fish Out: The following is almost an exact repeat of the advice given eating out on previous days. First order simple, such as broiled fish with steamed vegetables and brown rice. Tell the waiter you want no sauce, no gravy, nothing added. Then, knowing your calorie objective, and that fish is about 50 Calories per ounce, most steamed vegetable servings average approximately 50 Calories per cup, and rice is about 100 Calories per ½ cup, decide how much to eat – and take the remainder home. If fresh fruit is not an option, pass on dessert and have the evening snack specified for that day in the diet.

In a restaurant, some nutritionists recommend you eat the low-calorie items on your plate first. Start with the salad, soup and veggies. By the time you get to the fish and starches you will hopefully be full enough to be content with smaller portions of the higher-calorie choices.

<u>**Diet Tip of the Day:**</u> A handful of studies suggest that chewing gum may help reduce your craving for sweet snacks, and cut your caloric intake by about 50 per day. Another study actually showed that gum chewers experienced a small increase in their daily energy expenditure. And gum adds hardly any calories to your diet. Regular gum has about 10 calories and sugar-free varieties about five calories per stick.

<h1 style="text-align:center">Day 60 - Recipe</h1>

<u>Chicken Stew over Rice</u>

    4   boneless skinless chicken breasts (about 1 lb)
    1   medium Onion
    3   stalks celery
    12   mushrooms
    2   cups baby carrots
    3   cups broccoli florets
    ½   teaspoon black pepper
    ¼   teaspoon herb seasoning blend
    2   teaspoons Worcestershire Sauce
    1   bay leaf
    1   cup Cream of Chicken Soup (Campbell's)

Prepare a large, heavy, stove-top pot with cooking spray. Sauté at medium-high heat finely chop onion until caramelized. Cut chicken into bite size pieces and add to pot. Cook and toss until chicken is no longer pink. Add black pepper, herb seasoning and Worcestershire sauce. Stir. Add sliced celery and mushrooms, and then broccoli, carrots and bay leaf. Pour in Cream of Chicken soup. Gradually add one cup water while stirring. (You may want to add more water to get consistency desired.) Simmer until hot and flavors have combined. Serve over rice.

<u>Serves 4.</u> 360 Calories per serving (not including the brown rice below the stew).

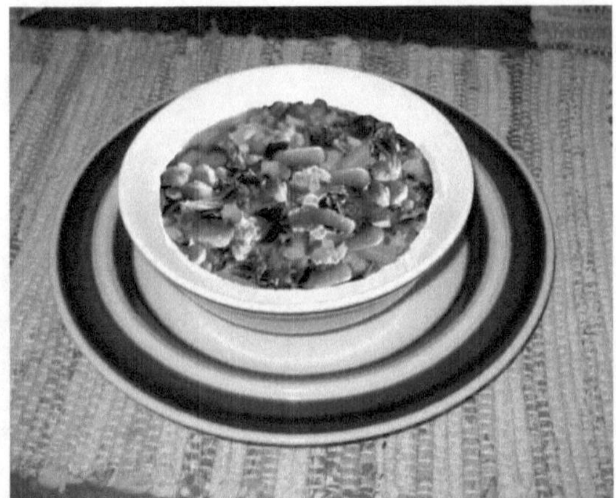

<u>Diet Tip of the Day:</u> Studies show people who eat 5 to 6 **mini-meals** and snacks a day don't feel as hungry and are better able to control their appetite and their weight.

Day 61 - Recipe

<u>Shrimp over Spaghetti</u>

- ½ lb spaghetti
- 1 lb shrimp, peeled and de-veined
- 6 ounces dry white wine
- 3 tablespoons olive oil
- 3 cloves garlic, sliced thin
- ¼ cup chopped basil leaves

Cook spaghetti according to package directions. Save ½ cup of the pasta cooking water.

In a large skillet over medium heat, cook olive oil and garlic, stirring until garlic turns golden, and then discard garlic. Add shrimp and increase heat to medium-high and stir in chopped basil leaves, white wine and ½ cup cooking water. Cook another 2 to 3 minutes or until shrimp are just firm. Spoon shrimp and sauce over spaghetti. Season with salt and black pepper. Garnish with parsley.

<u>Serves 4</u>. 450 Calories per serving

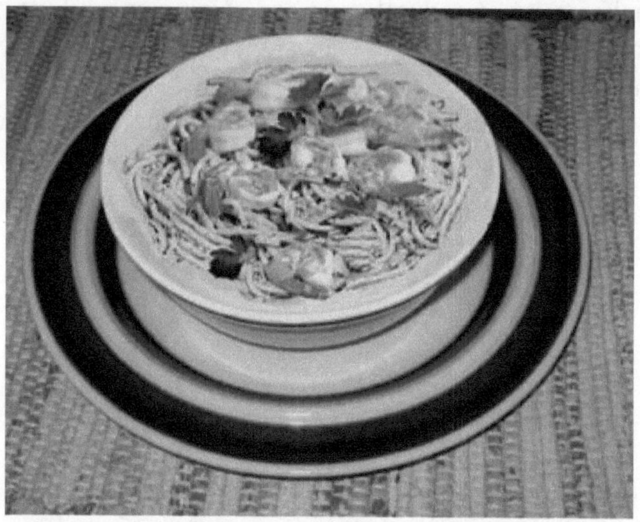

<u>Diet Tip of the Day:</u> If your caloric intake on a weight-loss diet is constant, your **rate of weight loss will decrease with time**. So if you want to lose weight at a constant rate over time, you must eat slightly less (or exercise harder) as you lose weight.

Day 62 - Recipe

<u>Beef Burgundy</u>

- 1 lb boneless beef chuck, trimmed & cut in 1" pieces
- 2 large carrots, cut into 1-inch pieces
- 1 medium onion, cut into 1-inch pieces
- 1 tablespoon flour
- 1 tablespoon tomato paste
- 1 clove garlic, crushed
- 1 tablespoon olive oil
- 1 cup dry red wine
- 2 sprigs fresh thyme
- 10 ounces mushrooms, sliced in half
- 8 ounces frozen peas

In Dutch oven, heat oil on medium-high until hot. Add beef and cook 5 to 6 minutes or until beef is browned on all sides. Transfer beef to a bowl. Preheat oven to 325° F. To drippings in Dutch oven, add carrots, garlic, and onion. Stir occasionally and cook 10 minutes or until vegetables are browned and tender. Stir in flour, tomato paste, ½ teaspoon salt, and ¼ teaspoon black pepper, and cook another minute. Add wine and heat to boiling, stirring until browned bits are loosened from bottom of Dutch oven. Return meat and any juices in the bowl to Dutch oven. Add thyme and mushrooms; bring to a boil. Cover and bake 1½ hours or until meat is fork-tender. Discard thyme sprigs. Before stew is done, cook peas per package instructions and add peas to Dutch oven.

<u>Serves 4</u>. 350 Calories per serving

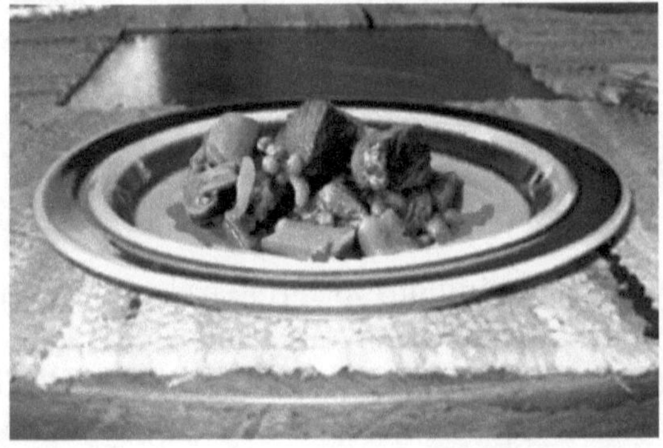

<u>Diet Tip of the Day:</u> When on a diet **simple is better**. Why? Because simple, uncomplicated meals usually contain fewer "hidden calories" than more elaborate dishes.

Day 63 - Recipe

<u>Chicken Cutlet</u>

Buy 4 skinless, boneless chicken cutlets or breast halves (about 1 lb), flattened to about ¼ to ½-inch thick.

- ¾ cup Panko bread crumbs
- ⅓ cup grated Parmesan cheese
- 1 egg, beaten
- 4 tablespoons extra-virgin olive oil, divided

Season chicken cutlets with salt and pepper. Combine bread crumbs and Parmesan cheese in a shallow bowl. Whisk egg in a separate shallow bowl. Dip chicken in egg and then coat both sides in crumb mixture.

Heat 2 tablespoons of olive oil in large skillet over medium-high heat. Add 2 cutlets, and cook 2 minutes on each side or until cooked through. Repeat with 2 tablespoons olive oil and remaining 2 cutlets. Serve hot.
<u>Serves 4.</u> 450 Calories per serving (chicken cutlet only)

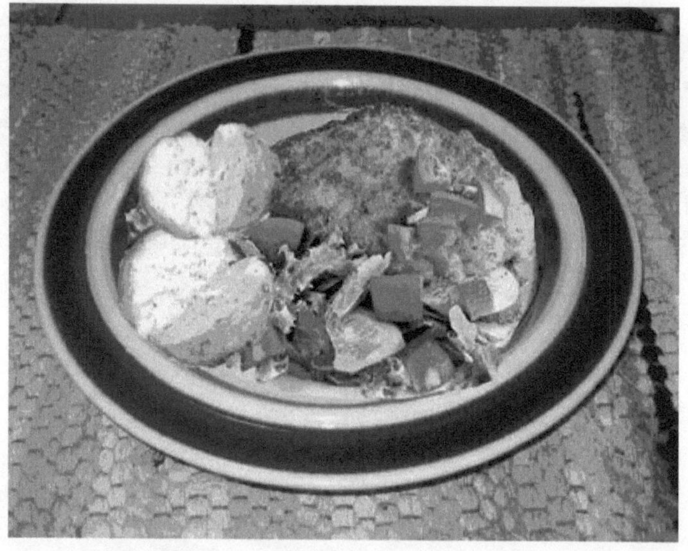

<u>Diet Tip of the Day</u>: **Working out at home** has some significant advantages. Your workout takes less time because you don't have to drive back and forth to a fitness facility; and you have the flexibility of dividing your workout into small time segments to fit your day, and working out at home is less expensive.

<u>Turkey Meat Loaf</u>

- 1½ cups finely chopped onion
- 1 tablespoon minced garlic
- 1 teaspoon olive oil
- 1 medium carrot, cut into ¼-inch pieces
- ¾ pound cremini mushrooms, finely chopped
- 1 teaspoon salt & ½ teaspoon black pepper
- 1½ teaspoons Worcestershire sauce
- ⅓ cup fresh parsley, finely chopped
- ¼ cup plus 1 tablespoon ketchup
- 1 cup fresh bread crumbs
- ⅓ cup 1% milk
- 1 whole large egg, & large egg white, lightly beaten
- 1¼ pound ground turkey (mostly light meat)

Preheat oven to 400°F. Cook onion and garlic in oil in a 12-inch nonstick skillet over moderate heat, stirring, until onion is softened, about 2 minutes. Add carrot and cook, stirring, until softened, about 3 minutes. Add mushrooms, ½ teaspoon salt, and ¼ teaspoon pepper and cook, stirring occasionally, until mushrooms are very tender, 10 to 15 minutes. Stir in Worcestershire sauce, parsley, and 3 tablespoons ketchup. Transfer vegetable mixture to a large bowl and cool.

Stir together bread crumbs and milk in a small bowl and let stand 5 minutes. Stir in egg and egg white, then add to vegetable mixture. Add turkey and remaining ½ teaspoon salt and ¼ teaspoon pepper to vegetable mixture and mix well. (Mixture will be very moist.)

Form into a 9 x 5-inch oval loaf in a lightly oiled 13 x 9 x 2-inch metal baking pan and brush meat loaf evenly with remaining 2 tablespoons ketchup. Bake in middle of oven until thermometer inserted into meat loaf registers 170°F, about 50 to 55 minutes. Let meat loaf stand 5 minutes. **<u>Serves 6</u>**. 240 Calories per serving

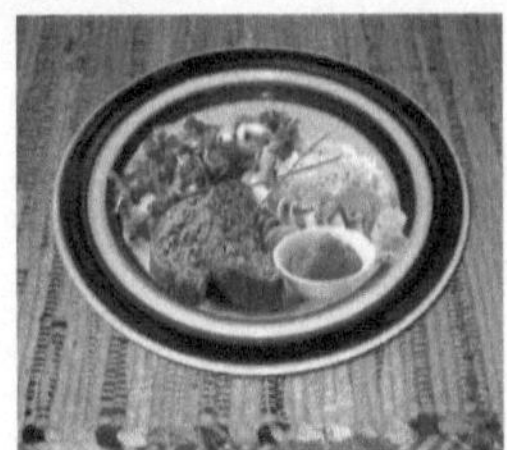

Photo shows meat loaf with noodles & mixed greens.

<u>Frozen-Fish Dinner</u>

No recipe today. No cooking today. It's your day off! To find a frozen fish dinner, please go to Appendix A (page 198) which lists approximately 150 frozen dinners manufactured by Healthy Choice, Lean Cuisine and Smart Ones.

Perusing the list, it is obvious that there are not many frozen fish dinners for sale at supermarkets. Note that if you do not use all of the **340 Calories allocated for this Day 5 meal**, use the excess calories anyway you wish. Splurge on extra dessert or save the calories for the next day and have a larger piece of pizza!

Please read the important **Frozen-Food Safety Warning** in Appendix B on page 204.

<u>**Diet Tip of the Day:**</u> **Muscle** is active tissue, fat is not. The more muscle you have, the more calories you burn. Muscle uses a significant number of calories every day for repair and rebuilding, giving your metabolism a boost even when you're resting. So make sure strengthening exercises (like weight lifting) are part of your workout.

<u>Pita Pizza</u>

  6 pita bread loaves (Joseph's Flax, Oat Bran & Whole Wheat Pita Bread -
  8 oz pkg)
  ¾ cup part-skim shredded mozzarella, divided
  1 large red pepper, sliced
  1 medium onion, sliced
  6 medium mushrooms, sliced
  ¾ cup tomato sauce, divided
  4 tablespoons olive oil

Cook olive oil in large skillet over medium-high heat. Add pepper slices,
onion slices and mushroom slices and sauté until they softened.

Toast pita loaves slightly (so they don't get soggy when sauce is
applied). Coat one side of pita with tomato sauce. Arrange pepper, onion and
mushroom slices on individual pita loaves and sprinkle shredded mozzarella
cheese on top.

In oven preheated to 400ºF, place pita loaves on baking tin coated with
cooking spray. Cook approximately 5 minutes or until cheese melts. Season
with salt and pepper to taste.

<u>Serves 3</u>. 430 Calories per serving (Two Pita Pizzas per serving.)

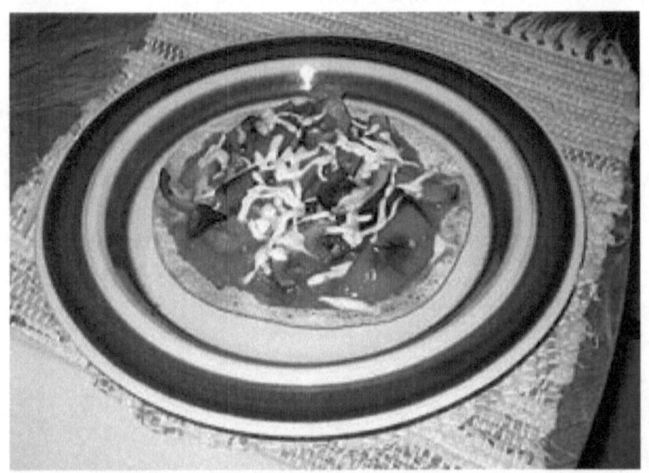

Note only one pita pizza shown. Serving size is <u>two</u> pita pizzas.

<u>**Diet Tip of the Day:**</u> On a reducing diet, **when you lose – you win**! You
win a much better chance for a longer healthier life, you win a sense of well-
being, you win a more attractive appearance – and finally you win a feeling
of accomplishment.

Day 67 - Recipe

<u>Chicken Dinner - Out</u>

No recipe today. No cooking today. Have a chicken dinner at your favorite restaurant, but make sure you choose a restaurant where you have a fighting chance to achieve your calorie goal. For your chicken dinner out, your maximum allowable calories (includes appetizer, soup, main course and dessert) are as follows:
- For **1,200 Calorie Diet**: 530 Calories
- For **1,500 Calorie Diet**: 630 Calories

Tips for Eating Chicken Out: First, order simple and order skinless white meat only, such as broiled chicken breast with steamed vegetables and brown rice. Tell the waiter you want no sauce, no gravy, nothing added. Then, knowing your calorie objective, and that chicken is about 50 Calories per ounce, most steamed vegetable servings average approximately 50 Calories per cup, and rice is about 100 Calories per ½ cup, decide how much to eat – and take the remainder home. If fresh fruit is not an option, pass on dessert and have the evening snack specified for that day in this diet.

In a restaurant, some nutritionists recommend you eat the low-calorie items on your plate first. Start with the salad, soup and veggies. By the time you get to the chicken and starches you will hopefully be full enough to be content with smaller portions of the higher-calorie choices. (Incidentally, feel free to substitute skinless white meat turkey for chicken.)

Finally, some dieticians advise their dieting clients not to eat out. That's right. They believe eating at home is safer. But our thought is you have to eat out eventually so why not learn how while your resolve is high?

<u>Diet Tip of the Day:</u> When you're eating out, consider **ordering children's portions** or a small sandwich as a way to trim calories and get the size of your meals under control.

Pork Medallions in Lime Sauce

- 1   pound pork tenderloin
- ⅓   cup all purpose flour
- 2   tablespoons olive oil
- 1   tablespoon unsalted butter
- ½   cup of white wine
- ¼   cup lime juice
- 2   stalks celery, chopped
- 1   medium onion, chopped

Trim away the thin silver skin on the tenderloin and all visible fat. Discard trimmings. Cut tenderloin into ½ to ¾ inch thick medallions. Sprinkle medallions with salt and pepper. Place flour in a shallow dish and coat pork medallions. Warm olive oil in a large skillet over medium-low heat. Working in batches if necessary, cook pork medallions, turning once, until well browned on both sides, about 5 minutes total. (Note internal pork temperature should be 160º F.) Transfer pork to a plate.

Add the wine and lime juice to skillet and bring to boil, scraping up browned bits from bottom of pan with wooden spoon and stirring occasionally, until thickened, about 4 minutes. Remove from heat; stir in butter, chopped celery and onion. Return pork to pan and warm though, turning medallions to coat with sauce.

Serves 4. 450 Calories per serving (pork medallions and sauce only)

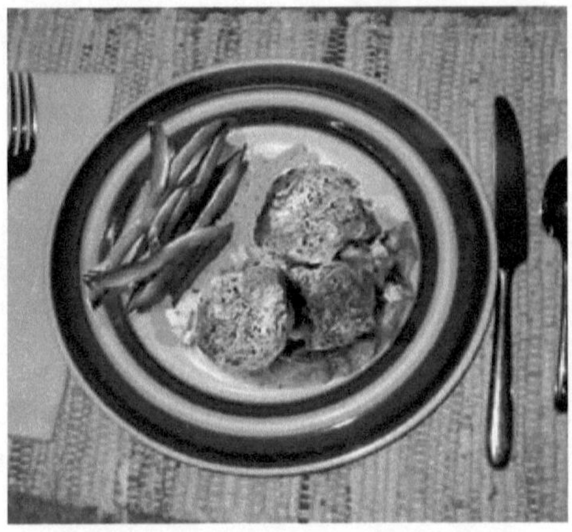

Diet Tip of the Day: Protein and carbohydrates are about 4 Calories per gram (110 Calories per ounce) and fat is 9 Calories per gram (260 Calories per ounce).

Healthy Chicken Salad

4	skinless, boneless chicken breast halves, cooked
2	beefsteak tomatoes, cut into large pieces
1	celery heart, chopped
¼	pound roasted red peppers, from jar, chopped
1	small red onion, peeled, halved
10	black olives, halved
1	small bunch basil, leaves only
1½	tablespoons red wine vinegar
3	tablespoons extra-virgin olive oil
¼	pound croutons

Shred cooked chicken and mix with croutons, tomatoes, celery, roasted peppers, red onion, olives and basil in large bowl and season with salt and black pepper. Drizzle with 3 tablespoons extra-virgin olive oil and balsamic vinegar and toss.

Serves 4. 330 Calories per serving

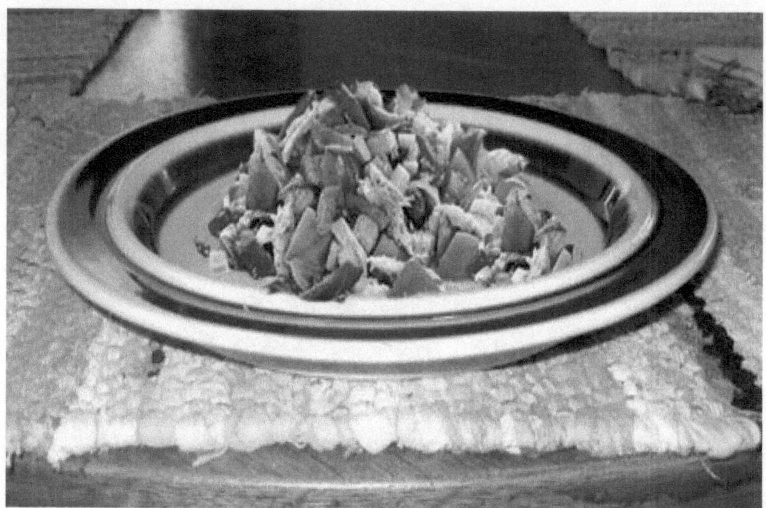

Diet Tip of the Day: In the view of many nutritionists, if you can afford it, buy local and **organic** but you don't have to buy organic across the board because not all organic-labeled products offer added health value.

Baked Cod

   4 cod fish fillets (4 to 5 ounces each)
   2 tablespoons flour
   2 tablespoons cornmeal
   2 tablespoons minced fresh herbs
   2 teaspoons lemon juice

Sprinkle cod with lemon juice. Mix flour, cornmeal and herbs and dust the cod with the cornmeal-herb mixture. Bake in oven at 375 ºF for 10 minutes. Add salt and black pepper to taste.
Serves 4. One serving is 230 Calories (cod only).

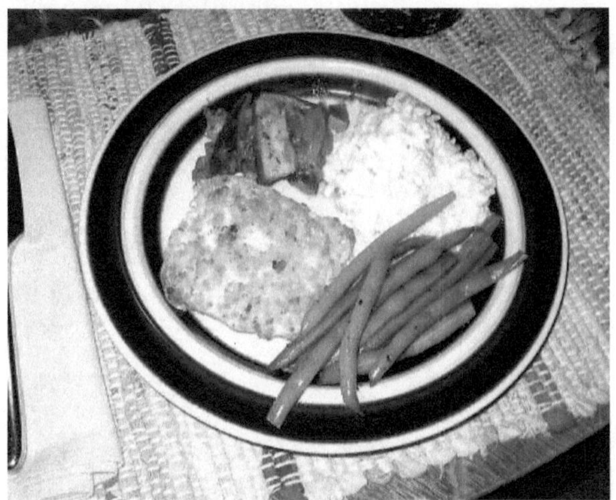

Diet Tip of the Day: It's worth **buying organic** for the "dirty dozen": peaches, strawberries, nectarines, apples, spinach, celery, pears, sweet bell peppers, cherries, potatoes, lettuce, and imported grapes. These fragile fruits and vegetables often require more pesticides to fight off bugs.

Day 71 - Recipe

Chicken Scaloppini

- 4 skinless, boneless 6-oz chicken breast halves
- 2 teaspoons fresh lemon juice
- ⅓ cup Italian-seasoned breadcrumbs
- ½ cup fat-free, less-sodium chicken broth
- ¼ cup dry white wine
- 4 teaspoons capers
- 1 tablespoon extra-virgin olive oil

Place each chicken breast half between 2 sheets heavy-duty plastic wrap and pound to about ¼-inch thick using meat mallet. Cut each breast in quarters. Brush chicken with juice, and sprinkle with salt and black pepper. Dredge chicken in breadcrumbs.

Heat a large nonstick skillet coated with cooking spray over medium-high heat. Add chicken to pan; cook 3 minutes on each side or until chicken is done. Remove from pan; keep warm.

Add broth and wine to pan, and cook 30 seconds, stirring constantly. Remove from heat. Stir in capers and olive oil – and serve immediately. **Serves 4**. 260 Calories per serving (chicken only)

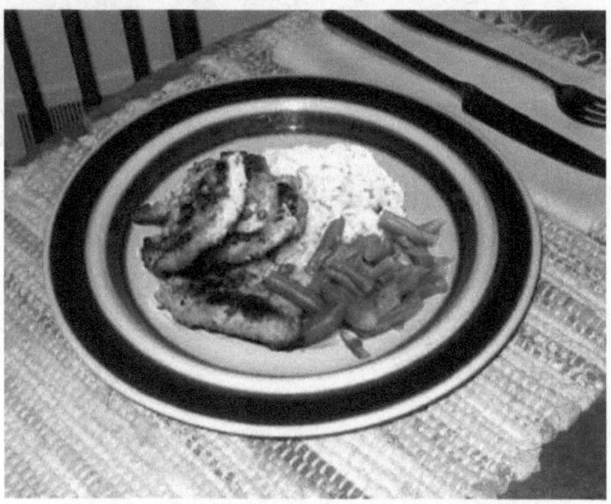

Chicken slightly burned, but still delicious!

Diet Tip of the Day: Nutritionists define a **"junk food"** as a food that offers little if any essential nutrients – except calories – and when eaten it replaces more important foods.

Day 72 - Recipe

Fish Dinner - Out

No recipe today. No cooking today. Have a fish dinner at your favorite restaurant, but make sure you choose a restaurant where you have a good chance to achieve your calorie goal. For today, your **goal for dinner is a maximum of 595 Calories**. This includes appetizer, soup, main course, dessert and wine.

Tips for Eating Fish Out: The following is almost an exact repeat of the advice given eating out on previous days. First, order simple, such as broiled fish with steamed vegetables and brown rice. Tell the waiter you want no sauce, no gravy, nothing added. Then, knowing your calorie objective, and that fish is about 50 Calories per ounce, most steamed vegetable servings average approximately 50 Calories per cup, and rice is about 100 Calories per ½ cup, decide how much to eat – and take the remainder home. If fresh fruit is not an option, pass on dessert and have the evening snack specified for that day in the diet.

In a restaurant, some nutritionists recommend you eat the low-calorie items on your plate first. Start with the salad, soup and veggies. By the time you get to the fish and starches you will hopefully be full enough to be content with smaller portions of the higher-calorie choices.

Diet Tip of the Day: In the U.S., we consume more than 100 pounds of **sugar** per year per person, totaling an unhealthy, nutritionally empty, 500 Calories per day. This large intake of sugar leads to obvious ills, such as obesity and tooth decay.

<h1 style="text-align:center">Day 73 - Recipe</h1>

<u>Pasta Pomodoro</u>

Pasta Pomodoro (Italian for pasta with tomatoes) is typically prepared with angel hair pasta, olive oil, fresh tomatoes, and fresh basil. It's light, delicious and easy to make.

- ¾ pound angel hair pasta
- 1½ pints cherry tomatoes (about 45), halved
- 8 fresh basil leaves, chopped
- 4 cloves garlic, minced
- 2 tablespoons olive oil
- 4 Tbsp grated parmesan cheese

Cook angel hair pasta per package directions. Over medium heat, sauté the garlic in olive oil until it just starts to turn golden. Add tomatoes and cook for about 10 minutes, or until they just start to release juices. Turn off the heat and stir basil into the sauce. Over the cooked pasta, spoon the tomato sauce with a little of the pasta water and garnish with more basil and grated cheese.

<u>Serves 4</u>. 420 Calories per serving

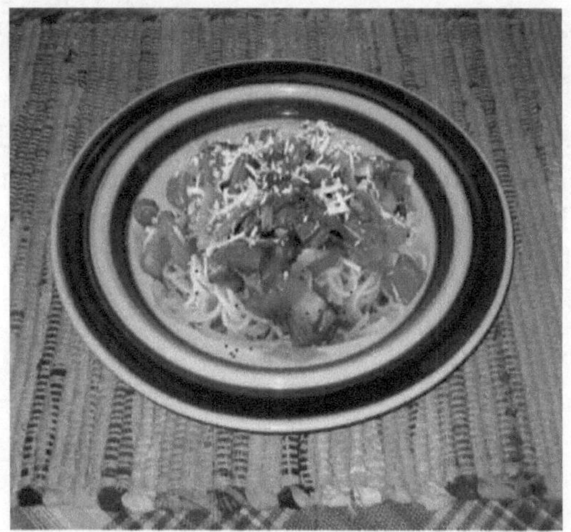

Above prepared with mix of cherry and plum tomatoes.

<u>**Diet Tip of the Day:**</u> Thinking about using **honey** rather than sugar? Honey has about 21 calories per teaspoon while sugar has 15. And the vitamin and mineral content of honey is very low.

180

Frozen Chicken Dinner

No recipe today. No cooking today. It's your day off! To find a frozen chicken dinner entrée please go to Appendix A (page 198) which lists approximately 150 frozen dinners manufactured by Healthy Choice, Lean Cuisine and Smart Ones.

Note that if you do not use all of the **300 Calories allocated for the Day 56 frozen dinner**, use the excess calories anyway you wish. Splurge on extra dessert or save the calories for another day.

Please read the important **Frozen-Food Safety Warning** in Appendix B on page 204.

<u>**Diet Tip of the Day:**</u> Many health care professionals think that eating a healthy **vegetarian diet** is one of the best things you can do for your short-term and long-term health. But a vegetarian diet must be carefully planned.

<u>Mediterranean Chicken</u>

4 small boneless skinless chicken breasts (about 1 lb total)
1 tablespoon paprika
1 tablespoon olive oil
½ teaspoon snipped fresh rosemary
2 cloves garlic, minced
¼ teaspoon ground black pepper
¼ cup dry red wine
3   tablespoons balsamic vinegar

Place chicken breast halves between two pieces of plastic wrap and pound with the flat side of a meat mallet into a rectangle ¼ to ½ inch thick. In a small bowl, combine paprika, oil, rosemary, garlic, and pepper; mixing well until it becomes a paste. Rub both sides of each chicken breast with paste mixture. Coat a 13x9x2-inch baking pan with nonstick cooking spray. Place coated chicken in prepared pan; cover and refrigerate for 2 to 6 hours.

Preheat oven to 450ºF. Drizzle chicken with wine. Bake for 6 to 8 minutes or until the chicken is no longer pink and a meat thermometer inserted in the thickest portion of the chicken registers 170ºF and the juices run clear. Turn the chicken once halfway through baking.

Remove from oven. Immediately drizzle vinegar onto chicken in the baking pan. Transfer chicken to serving plates. Stir the liquid in the baking pan and drizzle over chicken. If desired, garnish with fresh rosemary.
<u>Serves 4</u>. 180 Calories per serving (not including spaghetti squash & green beans)

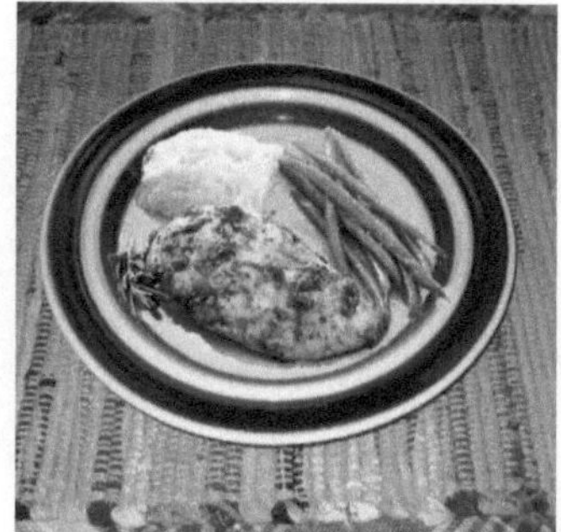

Photo shows chicken with spaghetti squash & green beans.

<u>Diet Tip of the Day:</u> Hunger is your body's way of telling you that you need calories. But **when you're done eating, you should feel better – satisfied but not stuffed**.

Day 76 - Recipe

<u>Gary & Sue's Grilled Scallops</u>

We were invited by our good friends, Gary and Sue, for dinner. They
prepared a simple, but nutritious low-calorie meal – which featured scallops.
(Scallops are a very low calorie food – expensive but great when you're on a
diet.) The photo below is our version of the main course they served that
night.

1½	pounds sea scallops
3	medium tomatoes, sliced, divided
4	ears of corn
2	tablespoons olive oil, divided
1	tablespoon balsamic vinegar, divided

Place scallops in a shallow bowl. Add olive oil and vinegar and toss to coat.
Grill scallops on medium-hot fire. Turn after two minutes or when first side
turns opaque. Grill until second side turns opaque – about another 2 minutes.
Don't overcook but test a scallop by cutting to make sure it's cooked through.
Salt and black pepper to taste.

<u>Serves 4</u>. The food pictured on the plate below totals about 360 Calories.

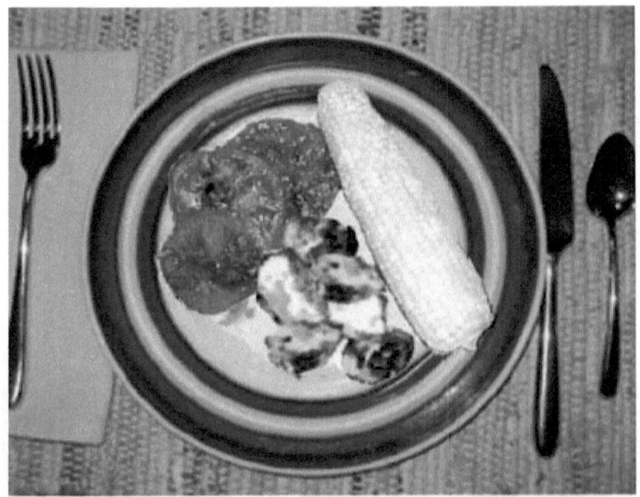

<u>Diet Tip of the Day:</u> When you eat fiber, it simply passes straight through,
untouched by but aiding your digestive system. **Zero calories absorbed!**

183

<u>Chicken with Peppers and Rice</u>

- 4   boneless, skinless chicken breast halves (about 1 lb)
- 1   red bell pepper, sliced
- 1   green bell pepper, sliced
- 1   yellow bell pepper, sliced
- 1   medium onion, sliced
- 1   ounce package of herb, garlic dip and soup mix
- 2   tablespoons olive oil
- ¾   cup wild rice, brown rice and wheat-berry mix.

Prepare wild rice per package directions. Cut chicken into 2 to 3-inch pieces. Place vegetables and chicken in re-sealable plastic bag. Add seasoning blend and olive oil. Seal bag and refrigerate for about two hours.

Preheat oven to 400°F. Place chicken and peppers in foil-lined baking pan. (Discard any remaining liquid in bag.) Bake 30 to 40 minutes, or until chicken is done. Broil an additional 2 to 3 minutes to brown chicken (optional).

<u>Serves 4</u>. 290 Calories per serving (Chicken, peppers and wild rice)

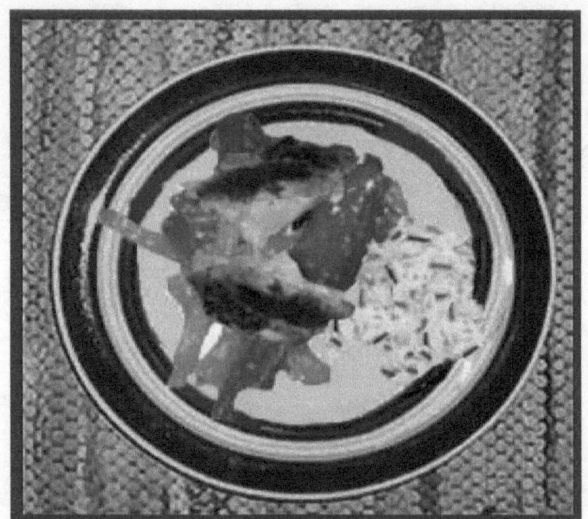

Chicken was browned too much but was still quite tasty!

<u>Diet Tip of the Day:</u> Most Americans consume too much sodium (salt). The U.S. Department of Agriculture Dietary Guidelines recommend that healthy adults **limit sodium intake to 2,400 mg per day**. (One teaspoon of salt contains about 2,300 mg of sodium.)

Day 78 - Recipe

<u>Trout with Lemon & Capers</u>

    4   trout fillets (4-oz each), skin attached
    3   tablespoons unsalted butter, divided
    2   tablespoons olive oil
    2   tablespoons lemon juice
    4   teaspoons chopped parsley
    1   teaspoon capers
    2   small lemons peeled and segmented

Score 2 crosswise slits (skin deep only) into each trout fillet using sharp knife. Turn the fillets over and season flesh with the salt and pepper.

Heat 1 tablespoon butter and the olive oil in a large nonstick skillet over medium-high heat. Place the fillets in the nonstick skillet, skin side up, and cook until golden brown, about 3 minutes. Turn and continue until cooked through and the skin begins to crisp around edges, about 2 more minutes. Transfer fillets to serving dish and keep warm.

Add the remaining 2 tablespoons butter to the hot skillet and cook until just brown. Stir in the lemon juice, parsley, capers, and lemon segments. Pour sauce over fillets and serve.

<u>Serves 4</u>. 340 Calories per serving (trout and sauce only)

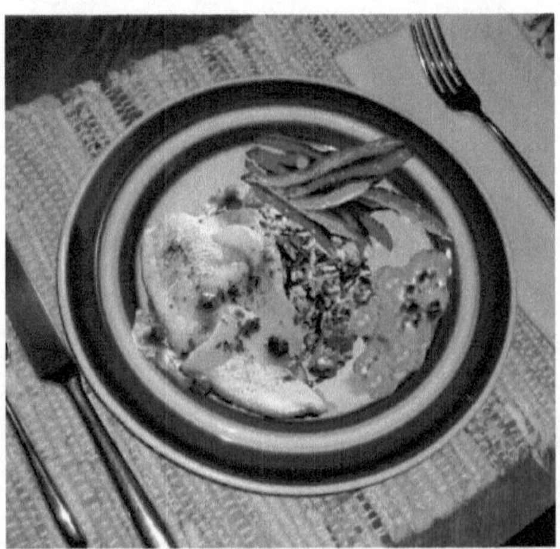

<u>**Diet Tip of the Day:**</u> Nearly every animal food, including dairy products, eggs, meat, poultry and fish are **complete proteins** because they contain all eight-essential amino acids. Soy is the only plant-based food that has all eight essential-amino acids.

Day 79 - Recipe

Italian Food - Out

No recipe today. No cooking today. Have dinner at your favorite Italian restaurant, but make sure you choose a restaurant where you have a reasonable chance to achieve your calorie goal. For today, **your goal for dinner is a maximum of 640 Calories**. This includes any appetizer, soup, main course and a 4 ounce glass of wine.

Tips for Eating Italian: You can consume a lot of calories in an Italian restaurant – if you order carelessly. For example a typical portion is often loaded with about 1000 Calories, then add another 100 Calories for a glass of wine.

First rule, order simple. Look for a dish with lots of vegetables, some fish or chicken. Then, knowing your 640 Calorie objective, and that chicken and fish are about 50 Calories per ounce, most steamed vegetable servings average approximately 50 Calories per cup, and pasta is about 200 Calories per cup, decide how much of the meal you can eat – and take the remainder the diet. Also see Eating Out (page 11) for more guidance.

Incidentally, although Italian is specified, feel free to substitute any other favorite ethnic food. Just make sure you don't exceed the maximum allowable 640 calories for this meal.

<u>Diet Tip of the Day</u>: Know your **daily caloric allowance** whether you are trying to maintain your weight or are on a reducing diet. (See "***Weight Control - U.S. Edition***" a NoPaperPress eBook where you can determine your daily caloric allowance using unique Weight Maintenance tables.)

Day 80 - Recipe

<u>Vegetable Chili</u>

 1 tablespoon olive oil
 2 medium carrots, cut into ½-inch pieces
 2 medium parsnips, cut into ½-inch pieces
 1 medium onion, chopped
 2 cans (15-ounces each) red kidney beans, drained
 4 teaspoons chili powder
 1 can (28-ounce) whole tomatoes in juice
 ¼ cup fresh cilantro leaves, chopped

In saucepot, heat olive oil on medium-high. Add carrots, parsnips, chopped onion, and cook 6 to 8 minutes or until all vegetables are tender and beginning to brown, stirring occasionally.

Meanwhile, on large plate, mash 1 cup drained beans. Stir chili powder into vegetables in saucepot; cook 1 minute, stirring. Add canned tomatoes with their juice, whole and mashed beans, and 2 cups water. Heat to boiling on high, breaking up tomatoes with spoon. Reduce heat to medium and cook, uncovered for 10 minutes, stirring occasionally. Finally, stir in cilantro and serve.

<u>Serves 4</u>.   360 Calories per serving

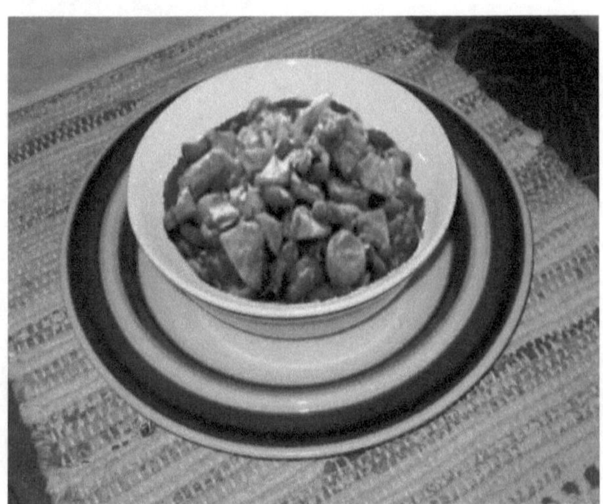

<u>Diet Tip of the Day:</u> **Carbohydrates** provide your body with its basic fuel, the energy your cells need to survive, as well as essential vitamins and minerals, fiber, and other beneficial compounds that promote good health.

Day 81 - Recipe

<u>Frozen-Meat Dinner</u>

No recipe today. No cooking today. It's your day off! To find a frozen meat dinner entrée please go to Appendix A (page 198) which lists approximately 150 frozen dinners manufactured by Healthy Choice, Lean Cuisine and Smart Ones.

Note that if you do not use all of the **300 Calories allocated for the Day 21 frozen dinner**, use the excess calories anyway you wish. Splurge on extra dessert or save the calories for another day.

Please read the important **Frozen-Food Safety Warning** in Appendix B on page 204.

<u>**Diet Tip of the Day:**</u> Keep low-calorie **lean sandwich fixings on hand** (whole-wheat bread, sliced turkey, reduced-fat cheese, lettuce, tomatoes and mustard).

Day 82 - Recipe

<u>Chicken Salad</u>

   4   skinless, boneless chicken breast halves (½ lb total)
   1   cup carrots, sliced
   1   cup red bell peppers, sliced
   4   green onions, diced
   1   cup edamame beans, cooked and shelled
   1   cup chow mien noodles
   2   hearts romaine lettuce
   4   cups mesclun mix or spring mix

<u>Salad dressing</u>: In a jar with a tight-fitting lid combine 2 tsp garlic powder, 1 tsp dried parsley, 1 tsp dried basil, 1 tsp honey, 2 tsp soy sauce, 4 tsp sesame oil, 2 tsp Sriracha (hot sauce – optional), 4 tsp Dijon mustard, 4 tbsp olive oil, 4 tbsp rice wine vinegar and a dash of black pepper. Shake well and set aside.

Grill chicken breast halves and then cut them into small pieces.

In a bowl, combine romaine lettuce, mesclun mix lettuces (or spring mix), carrots, red bell pepper, green onions and edamame. Add the dressing and toss. Add chow mien noodles and chicken and toss again.
<u>Serves 4</u>. 440 Calories per serving

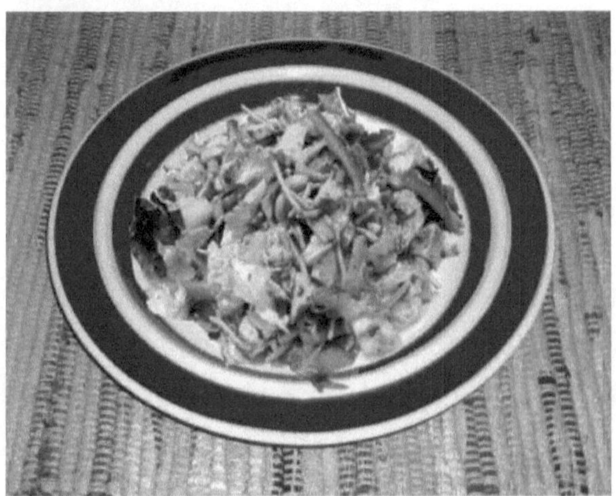

<u>Diet Tip of the Day:</u> Do not eat foods containing partially-hydrogenated vegetable oil because they are high in **trans fats**. This includes commercially prepared baked goods, snack foods, and processed foods, including most fast foods.

Day 83 - Recipe

<u>Hearty Lentil Stew</u>

- ½ cup chopped onion
- 2 garlic cloves, minced
- 1 tablespoon vegetable oil
- 1 cup lentils, rinsed
- 4 tsp vegetable or chicken bouillon granules
- 3 tsp Worcestershire sauce
- 1 bay leaf
- 1 cup chopped carrots
- 14.5-ounce can diced tomatoes with liquid
- 10-oz package frozen chopped spinach, thawed
- 1 Tbsp red wine vinegar

In a large saucepan, sauté onion and garlic in oil until tender. Add 5 cups of water, lentils, bouillon, Worcestershire sauce, ½ teaspoon salt, ¼ teaspoon black pepper and the bay leaf. Bring to a boil. Reduce heat; cover and simmer for 20 minutes.

Add the carrots, tomatoes and spinach; return to a boil. Reduce heat; cover and simmer additional 15 to 20 minutes, or until lentils are tender. Stir in vinegar and serve.

<u>Serves 4</u>. 260 Calories per serving

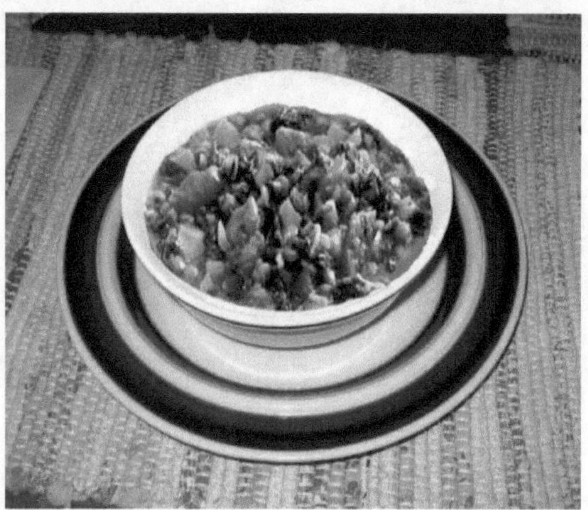

<u>Diet Tip of the Day:</u> Monounsaturated fats "**good fats**" are derived from plant sources, such as vegetable oils, nuts, and seeds. This type of fat is found in high concentrations in canola, olive and peanut oils.

Day 84 - Recipe

<u>Turkey Burger</u>

1¼	pounds ground turkey
1	tablespoon Worcestershire sauce
1	tablespoon chipotle mustard
1	tablespoon olive oil for brushing
4	seeded hamburger rolls

Lightly mix together the ground turkey, Worcestershire sauce, mustard, salt and black pepper. Form into 4 patties and brush each side lightly with olive oil.

Heat grill to medium-high. Place patties on grill and cook for 3 to 4 minutes each side for medium-well done. Salt and pepper to taste.
<u>Serves 4</u>. 355 Calories per serving (turkey burger only)

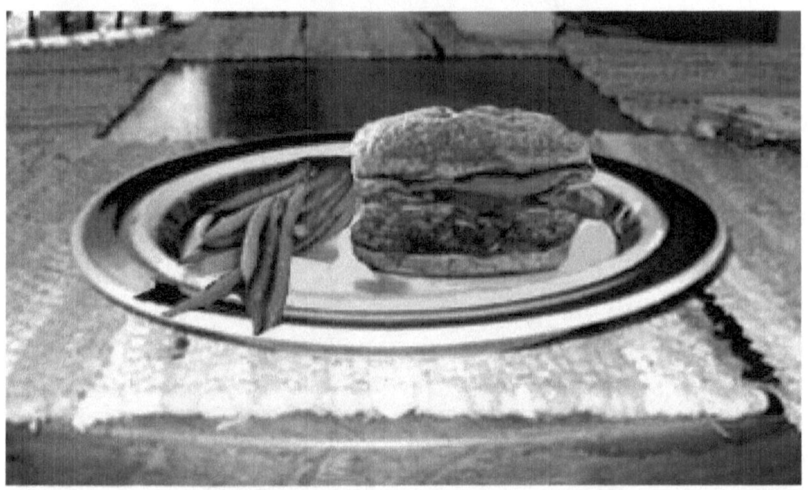

<u>Diet Tip of the Day:</u> Consistently **choose healthy foods**, avoid harmful foods and large portions and exercise regularly. Nothing else will control your weight over the long haul.

Day 85 - Recipe

Carrie's Low-Cal Meat Loaf

½ pound ground white meat turkey
½ pound ground beef (about 90% lean)
1 large egg
½ cup skim milk
¼ cup bread crumbs
¼ cup ketchup
¼ cup chopped carrots
¼ cup chopped onion

In a medium bowl, combine all ingredients. Add salt and pepper to taste.
Mix until blended and form into a loaf. Place loaf into oven preheated to 350
°F. Bake until an instant-read thermometer inserted in the center of the loaf
reads 160 °F. This should take about one hour.

Shown below is meat loaf, acorn squash (baked with 1 teaspoon of maple
syrup). Also shown is steamed spinach drizzled with extra-virgin olive oil.
Serves 5. About 290 Calories per serving (for meat loaf only). Note that
half a serving of left over meat loaf is to be eaten for lunch on Day 87.

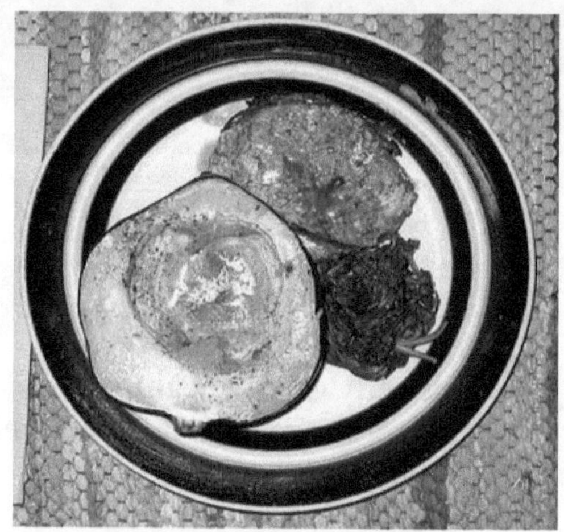

Diet Tip of the Day: Your **body weight fluctuates** two to three pounds
daily. Your body weight is lowest before breakfast and highest in the
evening before you retire.

<h1 style="text-align:center">Day 86 - Recipe</h1>

<u>Tuna & Bean Salad</u>

- 1   tuna steak, about 2 inches thick (14 ounces)
- 2   tablespoons extra-virgin olive oil
- 1   tablespoon lemon juice
- 1   garlic clove, crushed
- 1   tablespoon Dijon mustard
- 1   15-ounce can cannellini beans, drained
- 1   small red onion, thinly sliced
- 2   red peppers, seeded and thinly sliced
- ½   cucumber, halved lengthwise and thinly sliced
- 6   cups watercress

Heat a ridged grill pan coated with cooking spray over medium-high heat. Season tuna steak on both sides with coarsely ground black pepper. Cook the tuna 4 minutes on each side - the outside should be browned and the center light pink. Be careful not to overcook. Remove from the pan and set aside.

Mix together the oil, lemon juice, garlic, and mustard in a salad bowl. Season with salt and pepper to taste. Add the cannellini beans, onion, peppers, cucumber and watercress. Toss gently to mix. Cut tuna into ½-inch thick slices. Arrange on top of salad and serve with lemon wedges.
<u>**Serves 4**</u>. 355 Calories per serving

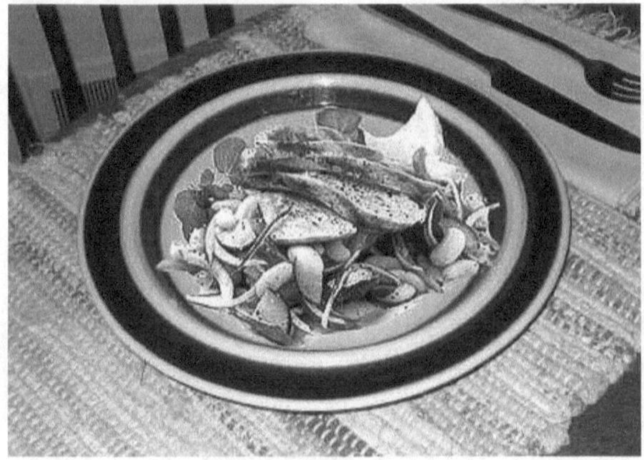

<u>**Diet Tip of the Day:**</u> In the United States, for a food to be labeled "**whole grain**" it must contain more than 51 percent whole grain by weight.

Day 87 - Recipe

<u>Pasta and Veggies</u>

¾ pound penne pasta
2 cups broccoli florets
1 red bell pepper, sliced
1 carrot, cut to 1-inch sticks
½ cup frozen green peas & ½ cup frozen sweet corn
1 small onion, chopped
1 tablespoon minced garlic
3 tablespoons olive oil
1 teaspoon fresh basil, chopped

Cook penne pasta per package directions. Drain and place pasta in a bowl. Pre-cook the carrot and broccoli florets.

In a large heavy skillet, heat the olive oil and sauté onion and garlic until lightly golden. Add vegetables and sauté until the peppers are soft. Combine sautéed vegetables in the bowl with the pasta. Toss well. Garnish with chopped basil, season to taste, and top with freshly grated Parmesan cheese. **<u>Serves 4</u>**. 460 Calories per serving

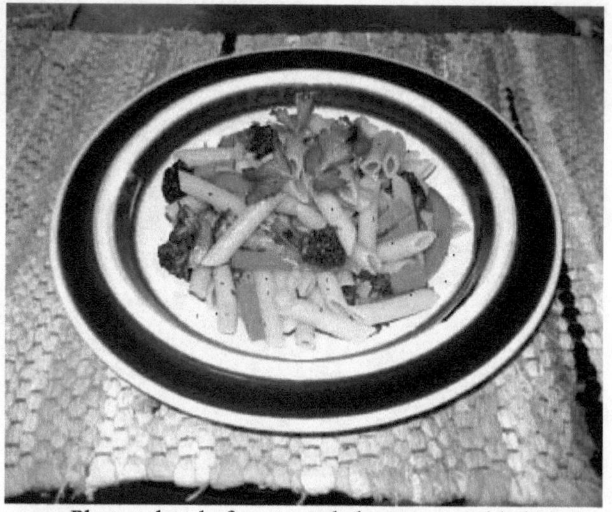

Photo taken before grated cheese was added.

<u>**Diet Tip of the Day**</u>: When possible, **select fresh and natural foods** and whole-grain products. Avoid chemical preservatives and additives, artificial and imitation foods, refined and processed foods, and foods that are comprised of "nutritionally-empty calories."

194

Day 88 - Recipe

Frozen Chicken Dinner

No recipe today. No cooking today. It's your day off! To find a frozen chicken dinner entrée please go to Appendix A (page 198) which lists approximately 150 frozen dinners manufactured by Healthy Choice, Lean Cuisine and Smart Ones.

Note that if you do not use all of the **300 Calories allocated for the Day 56 frozen dinner**, use the excess calories anyway you wish. Splurge on extra dessert or save the calories for another day.

Please read the important **Frozen-Food Safety Warning** in Appendix B on page 204.

<u>**Diet Tip of the Day:**</u> Understand that the only **sure way to slim down for keeps** is to eat less and exercise more. There are no safe short cuts or miracle methods for taking off weight.

Fish Stew

1	pound shrimp, peeled and de-veined
¾	pound skinless flounder fillet, cut into strips
1	pound new baby potatoes, halved
2	peppers (red and yellow) sliced into strips
1	onion, halved and sliced
4	ounces white wine
2	cups vegetable stock
2	cloves garlic, crushed
1	small bunch basil, shredded
1½	tablespoons olive oil

In a large pot, sauté garlic, onion and peppers in olive oil until they are completely softened. Stir in wine, vegetable stock and potatoes. Simmer until potatoes are tender.

Add the shrimp and flounder and cook for additional 4 minutes. Stir in basil and serve.

__Serves 4__. 300 Calories per serving

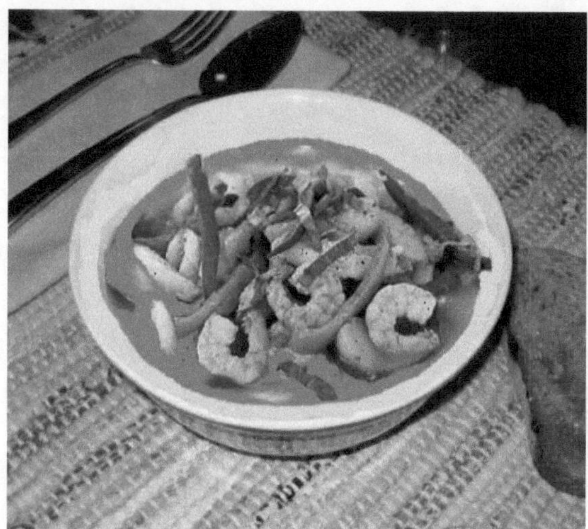

__Diet Tip of the Day:__ All **fish** are relatively low-calorie foods and are good sources of protein and fat-soluble vitamins A and D.

<u>Veal with Mushrooms & Tomato</u>

½ pound spaghetti
¾ pound veal cutlets
8   ounces sliced mushrooms
2   tablespoon olive oil, divided
2   tablespoons flour
3   green onions, small, sliced
½ cup chicken broth
14.5-ounce can diced tomatoes

Pound veal to about ¼-inch thickness. Rinse, pat dry and cut into 2-inch pieces. Heat 1 tablespoon olive oil in large nonstick skillet over medium heat. Add mushrooms and cook, stirring, until lightly browned. Remove and set aside.

Season veal with salt and pepper and coat lightly with flour. Add remaining olive oil to skillet and cook veal over medium heat for about 2 minutes on each side, or until browned. Add the green onions and cook for 1 minute longer. Add chicken broth and cook, uncovered, for 5 minutes. Add tomatoes; cover and simmer for 3 to 5 minutes. Serve over spaghetti cooked per package directions.

<u>**Serves 4**</u>. 520 Calories per serving (includes spaghetti)

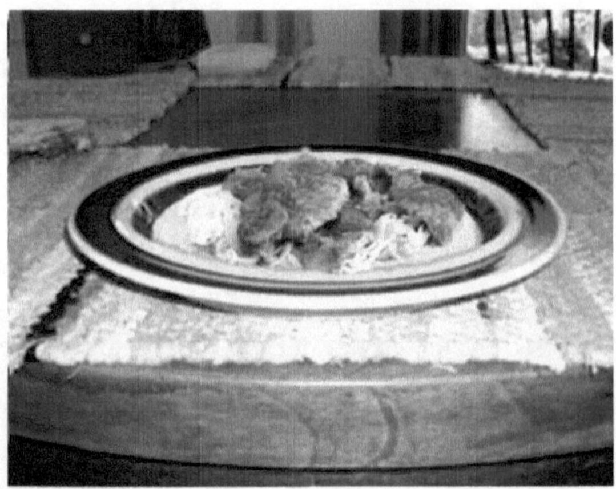

<u>**Diet Tip of the Day:**</u> Successful weight loss and subsequent weight maintenance **requires knowledge, desire and discipline**. Avoid the latest fad diets. Instead, take the time to develop a true understanding of weight control and then change your eating and activity habits accordingly.

Appendix A
Frozen Entrees

Appendix D lists three popular brands of frozen entrées: Healthy Choice, Lean Cuisine and Smart Ones. Note that each brand is color coded. The listing is further divided by entrée type: Poultry entrées, Meat entrées, Seafood entrées, Pasta entrées, Pizza and Other entrées. The entire table is arranged from the lowest to highest in calories. Note that the listed frozen entrées were available in most super markets as of 07/14/2020.

Entrée Type	Name	Brand	Calories
Poultry	Tomato Basil Chicken & Spinach	Smart Ones	160
Meat	Steak Portobella	Lean Cuisine	160
Meat	Asian Style Beef & Broccoli	Smart Ones	~~160~~ 170
Poultry	Herb Roasted Chicken	Lean Cuisine	170
Poultry	Slow Roasted Turkey Breast	Smart Ones	170
Poultry	Grilled Chicken Marsala	Healthy Choice	180
Poultry	Creamy Basil Chicken w Broccoli	Smart Ones	~~180~~ 170
Poultry	Garlic Chicken Rolls	Lean Cuisine	180
Meat	Beef Merlot	Healthy Choice	180
Meat	Homestyle Beef Pot Roast	Smart Ones	180
Poultry	Roasted Turkey & Vegetables	Lean Cuisine	190
Poultry	Chicken & Broccoli Alfredo	Healthy Choice	190
Poultry	Chicken & Vegetable Stir Fry	Healthy Choice	190
Other	Broccoli & Cheddar Roast Potato	Smart Ones	190
Poultry	Home Style Chicken & Potatoes	Healthy Choice	200
Poultry	Crustless Chicken Pot Pie	Smart Ones	~~200~~ 190
Poultry	Buffalo Style Chicken	Lean Cuisine	~~200~~ 190
Pasta	Angel Hair Marinara	Smart Ones	200
Poultry	Salisbury Steak	Smart Ones	200

Meat	Roast Beef & Mashed Potatoes	Smart Ones	~~220~~ 200
Pasta	Primavera Pasta	Smart Ones	210
Poultry	Honey Balsamic Chicken	Healthy Choice	210
Pasta	Ravioli Florentine	Smart Ones	210
Poultry	Cajun Style Chicken & Shrimp	Healthy Choice	220
Pasta	Cheese Ravioli Mushroom Sauce	Smart Ones	230
Poultry	Ranchero Chicken Wrap	Smart Ones	230
Poultry	Lemon Herb Chicken Picante	Smart Ones	230
Pasta	Cheese Ravioli Mushroom Sauce	Smart Ones	230
Meat	Meat Loaf with Mashed Potatoes	Lean Cuisine	~~230~~ 240
Seafood	Shrimp Alfredo	Lean Cuisine	~~230~~ 240
Poultry	Chicken Margherita	Smart Ones	~~220~~ 240
Poultry	Grilled Chicken Caesar	Lean Cuisine	240
Poultry	Honey Glazed Turkey & Potatoes	Healthy Choice	240
Pasta	Spicy Penne Arrabbiata	Lean Cuisine	240
Pasta	Four Cheese Cannelloni	Lean Cuisine	~~240~~ 250
Poultry	Creamy Basil Chicken w Tortellini	Lean Cuisine	~~240~~ 250
Pasta	Cheese Ravioli	Lean Cuisine	250
Pasta	Vermont Cheddar Mac & Cheese	Lean Cuisine	250
Pasta	Fettuccini Alfredo	Smart Ones	250
Poultry	Oriental Chicken	Smart Ones	250
Poultry	Fiesta Grilled Chicken	Lean Cuisine	250
Pasta	Chicken Linguini Red Pepper	Healthy Choice	250
Poultry	Golden Roasted Turkey Breast	Healthy Choice	250
Poultry	Chicken Mesquite	Smart Ones	250
Poultry	Chicken Oriental	Smart Ones	250
Poultry	Orange Sesame Chicken	Smart Ones	250
Poultry	Baked Chicken	Lean Cuisine	~~250~~ 260
Poultry	Teriyaki Chicken & Vegetables	Smart Ones	~~250~~ 260

Seafood	Tuna Noodle Casserole	Smart Ones	~~250~~ 270
Pasta	Spaghetti with Meatballs	Lean Cuisine	260
Poultry	Creamy Chicken & Noodles	Healthy Choice	260
Meat	Barbecue Steak w Red Potatoes	Healthy Choice	260
Pasta	Tortellini Primavera Parmesan	Healthy Choice	260
Pasta	Sesame Noodles with Vegetables	Smart Ones	~~260~~ 280
Pasta	Creamy Rigatoni w Chicken	Smart Ones	260
Pasta	Macaroni & Cheese	Smart Ones	260
Pasta	Butternut Squash Ravioli	Lean Cuisine	260
Other	Santa Fe Rice & Beans	Smart Ones	260
Other	Coconut Chickpea Curry	Lean Cuisine	260
Poultry	Glazed Turkey Tenderloins	Lean Cuisine	270
Poultry	Kung Pao Chicken	Healthy Choice	270
Poultry	Chicken Margherita w Balsamic	Healthy Choice	270
Poultry	Chicken Strips & Sweet Potatoes	Smart Ones	270
Pasta	Spaghetti with Meat Sauce	Smart Ones	~~270~~ 280
Meat	Salisbury Steak with Mac & Cheese	Lean Cuisine	~~270~~ 290
Pasta	Penne Rosa	Lean Cuisine	270
Poultry	Turkey Breast & Stuffing	Smart Ones	~~270~~ 280
Pasta	Classic Macaroni & Beef	Lean Cuisine	270
Pasta	Mushroom Mezzaluna Ravioli	Lean Cuisine	270
Pasta	Pasta with Swedish Meatballs	Smart Ones	~~280~~ 290
Other	Asian Pot Stickers	Lean Cuisine	280
Poultry	Sesame Stir Fry with Chicken	Lean Cuisine	280
Poultry	Roasted Turkey Breast	Lean Cuisine	~~280~~ 290
Poultry	Apple Cranberry Chicken	Lean Cuisine	280
Poultry	Chicken Fettuccini Alfredo	Healthy Choice	280
Poultry	Grilled Chicken Marinara	Healthy Choice	280
Poultry	Sweet & Spicy Orange Chicken	Healthy Choice	280

Poultry	Chicken Parmesan	Smart Ones	280
Poultry	Turkey Breast with Stuffing	Smart Ones	280
Meat	Beef & Broccoli	Healthy Choice	280
Meat	Meatball Marinara	Healthy Choice	280
Meat	Beef Teriyaki	Healthy Choice	280
Pasta	Spinach Artichoke Ravioli	Lean Cuisine	280
Other	Vegetable Fried Rice	Smart Ones	280
Pasta	Spinach Artichoke Ravioli	Lean Cuisine	280
Pasta	Linguini with Ricotta & Spinach	Lean Cuisine	280
Poultry	Chicken Fettuccini	Lean Cuisine	~~290~~ 280
Pasta	Spaghetti & Meatballs	Healthy Choice	280
Pasta	Spaghetti with Meat Sauce	Smart Ones	280
Other	Vegetable Fried Rice	Smart Ones	280
Other	Asian Pot Stickers	Lean Cuisine	280
Poultry	Chicken with Almonds	Lean Cuisine	290
Poultry	Chicken with Peanut Sauce	Lean Cuisine	290
Seafood	Shrimp & Angel Hair Pasta	Lean Cuisine	~~280~~ 290
Poultry	Grilled Chicken Pesto w Veggies	Healthy Choice	290
Poultry	General Tso's Spicy Chicken	Healthy Choice	290
Poultry	Pineapple Chicken	Healthy Choice	290
Poultry	Chicken Enchiladas Suiza	Smart Ones	290
Meat	Swedish Meatballs	Lean Cuisine	290
Seafood	Lemon Pepper Fish	Healthy Choice	290
Pasta	Pasta with Swedish Meatballs	Smart Ones	290
Other	Santa Fe Rice & Beans	Smart Ones	290
Pizza	Thin Crust Cheese Pizza	Smart Ones	290
Seafood	Parmesan Crusted Fish	Lean Cuisine	~~290~~ 300
Pasta	Santa Fe-Style Rice & Beans	Lean Cuisine	~~280~~ 300
Poultry	Roasted Turkey & Vegetables	Lean Cuisine	~~290~~ 300

Poultry	Sweet & Sour Chicken	Lean Cuisine	300
Poultry	Crustless Chicken Pot Pie	Healthy Choice	300
Poultry	Sweet Sesame Chicken	Healthy Choice	300
Poultry	Chicken Fettuccini	Smart Ones	300
Poultry	General Tso's Chicken	Smart Ones	300
Meat	Classic Meat Loaf	Healthy Choice	300
Seafood	Tortilla Crusted Fish	Lean Cuisine	~~300~~ 310
Pasta	Tuscan-Style Vegetable Lasagna	Lean Cuisine	~~300~~ 310
Pasta	Tortellini with Red Pepper Sauce	Lean Cuisine	300
Pasta	Broccoli Cheddar Rotini	Lean Cuisine	300
Pasta	Three Cheese Ziti Marinara	Smart Ones	300
Pasta	Lasagna Florentine	Smart Ones	~~310~~ 300
Seafood	Tortilla Crusted Fish	Lean Cuisine	~~300~~ 310
Pasta	Tuscan-Style Vegetable Lasagna	Lean Cuisine	~~300~~ 310
Poultry	Chicken Fried Rice	Lean Cuisine	~~300~~ 310
Poultry	Orange Chicken	Lean Cuisine	310
Poultry	Chicken Tikka Masala	Lean Cuisine	310
Poultry	Chicken Strips & Fries	Smart Ones	310
Poultry	Chicken Teriyaki	Lean Cuisine	310
Pizza	Thin Crust Pepperoni Pizza	Smart Ones	310
Pasta	Three Cheese Macaroni	Smart Ones	310
Pizza	French Bread Pepperoni Pizza	Lean Cuisine	310
Poultry	Chicken Spinach Mushroom Panini	Lean Cuisine	~~350~~ 310
Other	Spicy Beef & Bean Enchilada	Lean Cuisine	310
Poultry	Chicken Fried Rice	Healthy Choice	320
Meat	Sweet & Spicy Korean Beef	Lean Cuisine	320
Pizza	Farmers Market Pizza	Lean Cuisine	320
Pizza	Margherita Pizza	Lean Cuisine	320
Poultry	Chicken Carbonara	Lean Cuisine	330

Poultry	Mango Chicken w Coconut Rice	Lean Cuisine	330
Poultry	Country Fried Chicken	Healthy Choice	330
Other	Cheese & Fire-Roasted Tamale	Lean Cuisine	330
Poultry	Chicken Club Panini	Lean Cuisine	~~350~~ 340
Meat	Philly Style Steak & Cheese Panini	Lean Cuisine	~~330~~ 350
Poultry	Chicken Parmigiana	Healthy Choice	360
Poultry	Chicken Pecan	Lean Cuisine	~~320~~ 370
Poultry	Sweet & Sour Chicken	Healthy Choice	390
Pizza	Supreme Pizza	Lean Cuisine	~~330~~ 390

Increasingly, food giants like ConAgra, Nestlé and others that supply Americans with processed foods concede that they cannot ensure the safety of their food products. Frozen foods pose a particularly serious safety problem because unsuspecting consumers buy frozen foods for their convenience and incorrectly believe that cooking frozen foods is a matter of taste – not safety. Still the food industry says that extensive outbreaks of food-borne illness are rare, even though it is well-known that most of the millions of cases of food-borne illness every year go unreported or are not traced to the source. For example, each year approximately 40,000 cases of salmonella poisoning are reported in the United States – but perhaps as many as one million cases go unreported. (Salmonella is a type of bacteria most often found in poultry, eggs, unprocessed milk, meat and water.) Recently salmonella pathogens in some frozen meals have sickened thousands of people.

How could this happen? First, the supply chain for ingredients in processed foods – from flour to fruits and vegetables to flavorings – is becoming more complex and global in the drive to keep food costs down. As a result, government and industry officials concede that almost every food ingredient is now a potential carrier of pathogens. A further complication is that a large number of food companies subcontract processing work to save money and don't require suppliers to test for pathogens. In fact, companies often don't even know who is supplying their ingredients.

In addition, many frozen-food manufacturers have stopped cooking their products at high temperatures, a tactic they call the "kill step," which is intended to eliminate any lingering microbes. Frequently this process step turns some of the frozen food ingredients into mush. So, instead the "kill step" has been shifted to consumers. For example, ConAgra has added food safety instructions to its frozen meals, including the Healthy Choice brand. A typical "frozen-food safety" instruction offers this guidance: "Internal temperature needs to reach 165°F as measured by a food thermometer in several spots."

General Mills, now advises consumers to avoid microwaves altogether and cook their frozen pizzas only in a conventional oven. To be safe, always cook frozen foods so the internal temperature reaches 165°F.

Appendix C
Soup Selections

The following lists **canned** soup selections. See the important note at the end of list. The soup listed below were available in supermarkets as of 07/25/2020.

Soup	Calories
Progresso Chicken and Wild Rice	80
Progresso Hearty Chicken and Rotini	90
Progresso Garden Vegetable	90
Progresso Minestrone	110
Progresso Chickarina	110
Progresso Italian Wedding	120
Progresso Split Pea	130
Progresso Tuscan-Style White Bean	130
Progresso Lentil	140
Progresso Tomato Basil	150
Progresso Macaroni & Bean	160
Progresso Hearty Penne	160
Progresso Three Cheese Tortellini	170

* **Important:** When the Daily Meal Plan menu specifies soup, have only one serving (8 oz) unless stated otherwise. To improve the taste of canned soup, add a teaspoon of grated cheese before heating the soup in a microwave oven. After heating, add ½ teaspoon of olive oil. Stir and serve. These additions enhance the taste, and total about 30 Calories which should be added to the soup calories shown in the table above.

100-Day Super Diet-1200 Cal*	Weight Loss for Men - Metric*
100-Day Super Diet-1500 Cal*	Maximum Weight Loss- 1200 Cal*
100-Day No-Cooking Diet-1200 Cal*	Maximum Weight Loss- 1500 Cal*
100-Day No-Cooking Diet-1500 Cal*	Weight Control - U.S. Edition*
90-Day Smart Diet-1200 Cal*	Weight Control - Metric. Edition
90-Day Smart Diet-1500 Cal*	Prof Weight Control Women - U.S.
90-Day No-Cooking Diet - 1200 Cal*	Prof Weight Control Women - Metric
90-Day No-Cooking Diet - 1500 Cal*	Prof Weight Control Men - U.S.
90-Day Perfect Diet - 1200 Cal*	Prof Weight Control Men - Metric
90-Day Perfect Diet - 1500 Cal*	Weight Maintenance - U.S. Ed*
60-Day Perfect Diet-1200 Cal*	Weight Maintenance - Metric. Ed*
60-Day Perfect Diet-1500 Cal*	Weight Maintenance - UK Ed
50-Day Flex Diet-1200 Cal*	Weight Loss for Senior Men*
50-Day Flex Diet-1500 Cal*	Weight Loss for Senior Women*
30-Day Quick Diet - Women*	Eat Smart - U.S. Edition*
30-Day Quick Diet for Men*	Eat Smart - Metric Edition
30-Day No-Cooking Diet*	30-Day Mediterranean Diet
30-Day Diet - Women - Metric*	Exercise Smart - U.S. Edition*
30-Day Diet for Men - Metric*	Exercise Smart - Metric Edition
25 Day Easy Diet-1200 Cal*	Exercise Smart - UK Edition*
25 Day Easy Diet-1500 Cal*	Total Fitness - U.S. Edition
25-Day No-Cooking Diet	Total Fitness - Metric Edition
10-Day Express Diet	Total Fitness - UK Edition
10-Day No-Cooking Diet*	Total Fitness for Women-U.S. Ed*
7-Day Diet for Women*	Total Fitness for Women - Metric
7-Day Diet for Men*	Total Fitness for Women - UK Ed
7-Day No-Cooking Diets*	Total Fitness for Men - U.S. Ed*
90-Day Gluten-Free Diet-1200 Cal*	Total Fitness for Men- Metric Ed*
90-Day Gluten-Free Diet-1500 Cal*	Total Fitness for Men - UK Ed
30-Day Gluten-Free Quick Diet*	Senior Fitness - U.S. Edition*
30-Day Gluten-Free No-Cooking Diet*	Senior Fitness - Metric Edition*
7-Day Diet for Women - Metric*	Senior Fitness - UK Edition*
7-Day Diet for Men - Metric	Computer Diet - U.S. Edition*
7-Day Gluten-Free Express Diet*	Computer Diet - Metric Ed*
7-Day Gluten-Free No-Cooking Diet*	Reliable Weight Loss - U.S. Ed
90-Day Vegetarian Diet-1200 Cal*	101 Weight Loss Tips*
90-Day Vegetarian Diet-1500 Cal*	101 Healthy Eating Tips*
30-Day Vegetarian Diet*	101 Lifelong Fitness Tips*
7-Day Vegetarian Diet*	101 Weight Maintenance Tips
Weight Loss for Women*	101 Weight Loss Recipes
Weight Loss for Women - Metric	101 GF Weight Loss Recipes
Weight Loss for Women - UK	101 Veggie Weight Loss Recipes*
Weight Loss for Men*	30-Day Mediterranean Diet*
Maximum Weight Loss - 1200 Cal*	90-Day Mediterranean Diet - 1200 Cal*
Maximum Weight Loss - 1500 Cal*	90-Day Mediterranean Diet - 1500 Cal*

* These titles are available as both ebooks and paperbacks. Our ebooks are sold by Amazon, Apple, Google, Barnes & Noble and Kobo, but our paperbacks are only sold by Amazon.

Disclaimer

This book offers general meal planning, nutrition and weight control information. It is not a medical manual and the author does not claim to be medically qualified. The material in this book is not intended to be a substitute for medical counseling. Everyone should have a medical checkup before beginning a weight loss program. Moreover, the physician conducting the medical exam should be made aware of and should approve the specific weight control program planned. Additionally, while the author and publisher have made every effort to ensure the accuracy of the information in this book, they make no representations or warranties regarding its accuracy or completeness. Further, neither the author nor publisher assume liability for any medical problems that might result from applying the methods in this book, or for any loss of profit, or any other commercial damages, including but not limited to special, incidental, consequential or other damages, and any such liability is hereby expressly disclaimed.